Women's Health
Midwifery and Gynaecological Nursing

Christine Webb
BA, MSc, PhD, SRN, RSCN, RNT

Principal Lecturer in Nursing
Department of Nursing, Health and Applied Social Studies
Bristol Polytechnic

Edward Arnold
A division of Hodder & Stoughton
LONDON   MELBOURNE   AUCKLAND

© 1986 C. Webb

First published in Great Britain 1986
Second impression 1988

British Library Cataloguing in Publication Data

Webb, Christine
  Women's health: midwifery and
  gynaecological nursing.—(Using nursing
  models)
  1. Gynecologic nursing   2. Obstetrical
  nursing
  I. Title   II. Series
  618'.024613   RG105

  ISBN 0 340 36998 1

Typeset by Macmillan India Ltd., Bangalore. Printed and bound in Great Britain for Edward Arnold, the educational, academic and medical division of Hodder and Stoughton Limited, 41 Bedford Square, London WC1B 3DQ by The Eastern Press, London and Reading.

Women's Health

Midwifery and Gynaecological Nursing

USING NURSING MODELS SERIES

General Editors:

Susan E Norman SRN, DNCERT, RNT
Senior Tutor, The Nightingale School, St Thomas's Hospital, London
Computer Assisted Learning (CAL) Project Leader

Jane E Schober SRN, DIPN, RCNT, DNE
Associate Tutor, Royal College of Nursing (joint appointment with the Nightingale
School, West Lambeth Health Authority)

Christine Webb BA, MSC, PHD, SRN, RSCN, RNT
Principal Lecturer in Nursing, Department of Nursing, Health and Applied
Social Studies, Bristol Polytechnic, Bristol

Contents

Contributors

Sue Cowen SRN, SCM, RCNT, DIPN (LONDON) is Tutor, Women's Health, at St. Bartholomew's Hospital, London.

Marion McDonald SRN, SCM, DIPN, FETC works as a clinical teacher at North Tees General Hospital. She teaches on the obstetric module for RGN students.

Rosemary Methven MSc, SRN, MTD, DANS, RCNT is Senior Midwifery Tutor at the Birmingham Maternity Hospital. Previously she introduced the concept of the nursing process applied to midwifery care at Stepping Hill Maternity Hospital, Stockport, where she was also Senior Midwifery Tutor. She is a member of the editorial committee of *Midwives Chronicle* and the international journal *Midwifery*.

Christine Norton MA (CANTAB), SRN was until recently Senior Nurse (Continence Advisor) with Bloomsbury Health Authority, London. She was a founder member and first Honorary Secretary of the Association of Continence Advisors, and has lectured and written extensively on the subject of continence. Her most recent publication is *Nursing for Continence*.

Jo O'Neill MSc, BNurs, SRN, HV Cert, DN Cert is a Lecturer in Nursing at Bristol Polytechnic. She teaches students on the BSc (Hons) Nursing course, and is responsible for clinical placements. Before moving to Bristol, she was a Clinical Nurse Specialist at the Christie Hospital and Holt Radium Institute in Manchester.

Ann Webb SRN, SCM, NDN Cert, HV Cert is a practising health visitor in inner London. She helped to set up and is actively involved in the Hysterectomy Support Group.

Christine Webb PhD, SRN, RNT is Principal Lecturer in Nursing at Bristol Polytechnic. She is course leader to the BSc (Hons) Nursing course, and also teaches students preparing for the London University Diploma in Nursing, the Clinical Teacher's Certificate, and other nursing qualifications.

Preface

'Using Nursing Models' is the title of a series of books of which this is the first. The aim of the series is to foster a critical approach to nursing models and encourage nurses to experiment with them in their everyday work. The series is specifically aimed at specialist and post-basic students and practising nurses, and therefore builds upon basic knowledge by applying nursing research and theoretical ideas to clearly-defined areas of practice.

The phrase 'nursing must be a research-based profession' has become a slogan about which many nurses are sceptical when they note that the nursing process was introduced without being previously evaluated by means of systematic research. As nursing models are incorporated into nursing syllabi in the same untested way, practising nurses see yet another theory–practice gap in this inconsistency between rhetoric and policy.

The Using Nursing Models series is being developed in recognition of the need to analyse, criticise and evaluate the relevance of nursing models to standards of care. The format of each book is similar, with each chapter presenting a care plan for an individual patient and being based on a nursing model. Authors of individual chapters are specialist nurses who base their care plans on a solid research background in their particular field of expertise, and who discuss the wider implications of using models and the nursing process for nursing practice, management and education.

In this volume, experienced midwives and gynaecological nurses relate research, nursing models and the nursing process to the care of their women patients. In doing so, they draw in the sensitive topic of sexuality in nursing care and show how patients' or clients' individual needs and problems are linked with social definitions of femininity, health and sickness.

Writing the book has not been an easy task. The use of nursing models is a relatively new approach for all the authors, and they make no claims to be experts in this or to have all the answers. Their aim is to try to come to grips with the new ideas and to test them out in a tentative way, in order to see whether they are practicable and useful in improving the delivery and quality of nursing care.

My own interest in using nursing models began when I was appointed Chief Assessor for *Unit 3: The Application of Care* in the London University Diploma in Nursing. Writing a care plan based on a model is one item of assessed coursework in the Unit, and my attempts to grapple with nursing models were spurred on and enriched by having to 'moderate' over 400 of these care plans each summer. I would like to acknowledge the contribution this has made to my thinking, and to thank the Diploma in Nursing students who shared in what has been— for all of us, I am sure—a stimulating but at times painful experience! The exercise has helped to push forward the frontiers of nursing knowledge by raising our consciousness of the issues involved in using nursing models.

If this book succeeds in provoking more critical debate and encouraging others to 'have a go' at using the models, then its aim will have been achieved.

Christine Webb
Bristol, 1986

Note: Due to the need for confidentiality, a fictitious name and address are used in the care plans, and all midwives' signatures are omitted from the relevant documents.

Acknowledgements

I should like to thank all the authors of individual chapters for their willingness to take up the challenge which using nursing models presents to us all. Adapting to a new approach is far from easy, and they entered into the spirit of the venture enthusiastically and carried it through with great competence.

I am also grateful to Angela King for transforming my doodles into the elegant cartoons in Chapters 1 and 9.

I owe an enormous debt to Susan Devlin and Alison Fisher of Hodder and Stoughton for their interest, patience and hard work throughout the process of producing the book. They shared so fully in the enterprise that I feel confident that they would now be able to draw up care plans based on nursing models to satisfy the most demanding sister or tutor!

I

Introduction: towards a critical analysis of nursing models

Christine Webb

British nursing always seems to miss the boat. Salmonisation introduced a strongly hierarchical management structure to nursing when other management theorists had already passed on to more humanistic styles, and behavioural objectives were seized on as the answer to curriculum planning when other educationalists were rejecting them as too constricting and mechanistic. The nursing process was decreed to be the essential basis for direct nursing care by statutory bodies without any prior evaluative research to test its feasibility and relevance in this country. And now nursing models are appearing in basic and post-basic syllabi at the same time as many nurses in the USA are forcefully rejecting them after 10 years or more of struggling with their implementation in curricula and care planning (Webb 1984a). One reason for this rejection is that the

> viewpoints expressed in them were being strongly repudiated by a growing number of philosophers of science. In other words, nursing's theoretical link to philosophy was . . . . about a decade behind the times
>
> (Silva & Rothbart 1984:8)

Practising nurses themselves, therefore, must evaluate nursing models and their usefulness in patient care. This process will involve examining what is written about the models, assessing what the models say, and making judgements about their potential contribution to raising the quality of care, enhancing student learning, and adding to the professional and intellectual standing of nursing.

This chapter begins this dissection and evaluation by probing the origins of nursing models and their often hidden assumptions. It paves the way for more practical tests of their value in the following chapters, in which nurses discuss their attempts to use the various models in their daily work. The concluding chapter looks back over these efforts, identifies the benefits and difficulties which have emerged, and considers the lessons learned for future use and adaptation of the models in British nursing.

What is theory?

Theories, models, conceptual models, conceptual frameworks. . . . These are just some of the terms used to describe what, for simplicity's sake, we shall term 'models' in this discussion. The situation is further complicated because writers adopt different definitions of a theory, model, and so on, while others use the terms interchangeably. Examples of this varying terminology are illustrated in Figure 1.

If any common threads can be picked out from this confusion they are that theories are the most complex and systematically worked-out level of thinking, while models are simplified or diagrammatic representations. As Lancaster and Lancaster (1981) say:

> A model is a device to facilitate the examination and analysis of concepts . . . an approximation or abstraction of reality . . . attention is focussed only on the details of reality that are perceived to have the greatest relevance to the situation. (pp32-3)

A theory, however,

> must be precise and limited, and the concepts need to be clearly defined. (p33)

Thus, a model is a simplified version of reality,

Fig. 1.1   Some definitions of theories, models and conceptual frameworks

THEORY

Theory (takes) the form of concepts, principles, processes and the like, (and is used) to sharpen observations and to understand the phenomena within the domain of nursing practice. Such understanding precedes and serves as a basis for determining nursing actions to be taken.
(American Nurses' Association 1980)

. . . an organized set of concepts, definitions and propositions projecting interrelationship among concepts and providing a systematic view of phenomena in order to describe, explain, predict and/or control approaches to nursing practice.
(National League for Nursing 1983)

. . . a statement that purports to account for or characterize some phenomenon. A nursing theory, therefore, attempts to describe or explain the phenomenon called nursing. A theory is always a shorthand way to understand or characterize a phenomenon . . . In other words, it pulls out the salient parts of a phenomenon so that one can separate the critical and necessary factors (or relationships) from the accidental and unessential factors (or relationships). In this way a theory is like a map of a territory as opposed to an aerial photograph. The map does not give the full terrain, (ie the full picture); instead, it picks out those parts that are important for its given purpose.
(Stevens 1979)

A theory may be defined as a scientifically acceptable general principle which governs practice or is proposed to explain observed facts. Another definition of theory is that it is a logically interconnected set of propositions used to describe, explain, and predict a part of the empirical world . . . theory refers to the lawlike propositions of given phenomena within the model . . . Theories provide the theoretical basis for the model's view of the (situation).
(Riehl & Roy 1980)

A theory is a proposed explanation whose status is still conjectural in contrast to well-established propositions that are regarded as reporting matters of actual fact . . . . a set of interrelated concepts, definitions, and propositions that presents a systematic view of phenomena by specifying relations among variables.
(Thibodeau 1983)

MODEL

A model is defined as a way of presenting a situation in logical terms to show the structure of the original idea or object. It is a representation of the original idea or object that gives direction in much the same way that a dress pattern is a guide and provides instructions for making a dress.
(Rambo 1984)

A model can be defined as a symbolic depiction in logical terms of an idealised, relatively simple situation showing the structure of the original system. A model, then, is a conceptual representation of reality. This can be simply illustrated by examining a toy model of a car. Such a model is not actually a car, but its pieces represent the features of the actual car. These models display the outline or . . . . sketch of the original article.
(Riehl & Roy 1980)

CONCEPTUAL FRAMEWORK

A conceptual framework is a set of general ideas, or concepts, that are logically interrelated . . . The concepts are abstract ways of looking at the client, nursing goal, and nursing intervention . . . One's conceptual perspective on clients and on nursing's goals strongly determines what kinds of things one assesses. Everyone has a perspective, whether in conscious awareness or not. Problems can arise if the perspective 'in the head' is inconsistent with the actions taken during assessment. Information collection has to be logically related to one's view of nursing.
(Gordon 1982)

whose aim is to help us to understand a phenomenon such as nursing. A theory is more sophisticated and advanced because it includes definitions of all the concepts involved, and statements about how these are linked together. A model is a skeleton which is fleshed out by the details of a theory, while a conceptual framework is simply 'conjecture', undeveloped ideas or speculation (Menke 1983). Much time and effort, and indeed many entire books, have been devoted to discussions of the differences between a model and a theory, and whether various nursing 'models' fall into one category or another (see for example, Stevens 1979, Riehl & Roy 1980). Some recent writers consider that these efforts have generated more heat than light, and suggest abandoning this largely semantic argument in favour of attempts to use the models and systematically evaluate their intellectual and practical worth (Flaskerud & Halloran 1980, Hardy 1982, Meleis 1985).

There is clearly a need to follow this more pragmatic direction, and indeed this is a principal objective of the Using Nursing Models series. But the question of the status of nursing models should not be dismissed without considering why the theory-models-conceptual framework debate is important. Two major and linked reasons have been put forward for adopting nursing models. Firstly, if a profession is an occupation based among other things on the possession of a body of knowledge (Freidson 1977), then nursing could achieve full professional status comparable with medicine, law and so on, by basing its practice on these models (Lancaster & Lancaster 1981). Secondly, the quality of care given by such a profession would be higher because professional practice would be built on a systematic knowledge base (Hardy 1982).

If the future professional status of nursing is to depend on use of nursing models, then it is essential that their intellectual status matches up to that of theoretical thinking in other professions (Walker 1983). This is why it is essential for nurses to analyse the models critically and evaluate their status. If we base our profession on models which do not match up to those used in other professions, and which are judged by other

professionals to be inferior, then nursing will remain a 'semi-profession' or indeed no profession at all according to the definition of a profession widely accepted in sociological literature (Freidson 1970).

Nurses who have expressed doubts about the intellectual status and rigour of nursing models suggest that it would be better to use the term 'conceptual framework', because this terminology acknowledges the low level of development of theoretical thinking about nursing in relation to other disciplines. Adopting this term, they consider, will forestall embarrassing inter-professional comparisons from which nursing is bound to emerge with a diminished status. It also emphasises that we have a great deal of rigorous thinking and research to do before nursing comes anywhere near to developing true theories of or for nursing (Flaskerud & Halloran 1980, Kasch 1984, Webb 1984a).

This debate, however, is based on a restricted definition of 'theory'. It defines theory as 'scientific theory', which is:

> a systematically related set of statements, including some lawlike generalisations, that is empirically testable. The purpose of theory is to increase scientific understanding through a systematized structure capable of both explaining and predicting phenomena.
>
> (Lancaster & Lancaster 1981:33)

There are two problems with this definition of theory as 'scientific theory'. Firstly, it is based on a particular, restricted and increasingly challenged notion of science and secondly, there are many other kinds of theory which are equally valid ways of interpreting the world. Philosophical theory is derived from logical thinking, political theory considers policy decisions in terms of their implications for different social groups, and theological theory is developed from religious writings, revelations and 'evidence' of 'divine works' (Fowler and Fowler 1973). Therefore, many different kinds of theory exist, and the kind of scientific theory represented by most nursing models is but one of these. A theory is not necessarily inferior or of little practical value just because it does not stand up to scrutiny as a particular kind of scientific theory.

In order to delve further into this question of the status of nursing models and their usefulness in gaining professional standing and improving the quality of care, it is necessary to explore in greater depth their intellectual underpinnings.

What is Science?

'Real' science?

Most nursing models are designed to constitute 'a body of scientific knowledge characterised by descriptive, explanatory and predictive principles about the life process' (Rogers 1963:11) and to 'yield predictable (and desirable) responses in patients when implemented in patient care' (Johnson 1959:292).

Epistemology is the study of the philosophies and methods of thinking and studying which underlie a discipline, and one of its truisms is that these ways of thinking and methods of study are inseparable and interlinked. Particular kinds of ideas need particular methods for their study and research, and a certain kind of prescription for action also necessarily emerges from any theory developed in the course of study. In other words, theory and practice are necessarily and inevitably connected with each other. The kind of thinking lying behind nursing models which aim for explanation and predictable outcomes is called 'logical positivism', or simply 'positivism'. Fay (1975) characterises positivist science in the following way

> we understand a state of affairs scientifically only to the extent that we have the knowledge of what to do in order to control it, and it is thus that the ability to control phenomena provides the framework in terms of which scientific explanation proceeds. (p40)

Scientific knowledge, therefore, 'provides the basis for manipulative control', and what counts as scientific knowledge is 'that which gives us the means by which we can in principle control phenomena' (Fay 1975: 41). The methods of

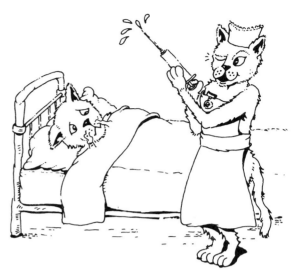

Time for your next dose of logical positivism, Mr Jones!

positivist science are said to be 'objective' because they use controlled observation and experimentation in order to verify explanations. This style of reasoning is often referred to as 'the scientific method' or 'the hypothetico–deductive method'. This means that a scientist starts off with a theoretical idea obtained from previous research, literature or observation, and formulates from this a hypothesis or testable idea. By a process of deduction, the scientist works out, or deduces, how the phenomenon to be studied will behave, and then proceeds to test the hypothesis by objective methods. If the hypothesis is confirmed, this will allow future occurrences of the same event to be predicted accurately. In other words, a law will be established which allows predictability and, if outcomes are predictable, then the way is opened for their control by humans. For example, if repeated, systematic and objective experimentation shows that a substance kills a certain bacterium with sufficient regularity, then that substance can be used to control infections. Positivist science is therefore defined by its ability to control phenomena.

Positivist science, and particularly positivist social science, can be criticised in a number of ways, however. Firstly, its 'objectivity' is in question because a scientist's personal values enter into the research process at many points. Deciding what to study in the first place is a very subjective matter which inevitably involves personal values; this is obvious when we consider that two identically qualified scientists may choose to carry out research into germ warfare or medical pharmaceutics, into agricultural pest control or organic farming, or into electroconvulsive therapy (ECT) or therapeutic communities. Throughout the research process, decisions about which line of investigation to pursue and how to do this are also made partly on the basis of personal preference, and when analysing the research findings this type of influence is again pervasive. Everyone knows by now that statistics can be used to prove anything the scientist wishes (Huff 1979), and the way certain findings are reported and others suppressed are also the result of individual values and preferences (Spender 1981). Thus, value-decisions are part and parcel of any kind of research, but this is not always acknowledged and discussed. The 'free-floating intellectual' who is above and untouched by particular values (Mannheim 1966) has long since been put to rest because of all this evidence that it is impossible for a human being to act or take any decision whatsoever without personal beliefs and values having an influence.

Another problem for positivist social science is that its 'data' are real people who are thinking and acting beings, and not passive objectives to be experimented upon and manipulated like substances in a test tube or iron filings around a bar magnet. In addition to ethical issues of how far it is morally acceptable to involve human beings in research, there is the problem that unique persons, by definition, do not all behave in the same way. If scientists assume that these 'units of data' are all equal and can be added, subtracted, multiplied and divided in statistical manipulations, they are misrepresenting what really goes on in social life, imposing their own definitions on other people, and indulging in 'measurement by fiat' (Cicourel 1964). A clear example of this occurred in a study of recovery from hysterectomy, in which women were pre-

sented with a list of 'mood adjectives' and asked to tick whether they experienced each mood 'not at all', 'a little', 'quite a bit', or 'extremely' (Webb 1984b). Several women asked the researcher whether the mood adjective 'worthless' meant 'not having much money', thus revealing how words are differently interpreted even by people from a single cultural background. By assuming that all the women were understanding the adjectives in the same way, and by using their scores to 'measure' their moods, the researcher was not objectively analysing data, but was in fact imposing her own assumptions on her interviewees. Examples are legion of how people's behaviour varies and is influenced by the very fact that they are being studied, the Hawthorne experiment being perhaps the most famous. In this study of worker motivation and productivity, it was found that productivity was increased merely because of the presence of researchers (Goode & Hatt 1952). Therefore, the fact that the 'data' observed by social scientists is fundamentally different from that of physical scientists makes the methods and assumptions of positivist or 'real' science extremely dubious.

'Soft' science?

Some early social scientists, notably Max Weber, quickly realised that positivist methods were inappropriate to the study of social life. They put forward as an alternative an 'interpretive' social science based on different assumptions and methods, and leading to different outcomes and implications for practice in comparison with the predictability and control of positivist science.

Interpretive social scientific methods are based on the assumption that 'subjective meaning', or the meaning an individual person gives to events and feelings, is valid data. Investigating social life scientifically in this version involves listening to what people say or observing what they do, and using empathic understanding and a 'sociological imagination' (Wright Mills 1959) to interpret their meanings. 'Proof' of the 'truth' of these interpretations then depends on whether the actors themselves accept them and not, as in positivist science, on whether they identify causes, predict outcomes and allow control (Fay 1975).

Interpretive social scientists do not start off with a theory and proceed to test it like positivists do, but instead they build up theory on the basis of what they learn from the people they study. This 'inductive' method of constructing theory grounded in the data (Glaser & Strauss 1967) contrasts with the hypothetico-deductive method which is often taken to be *the* scientific method.

The implications of interpretive social science for practice or policy are also different, and arise inevitably from this different methodology (Fay 1975). The logical consequence of placing primary emphasis on the meanings which individuals communicate to the researcher is that resulting social policy concerns itself with improving communications, clearing up misunderstandings, and changing people's ways of thinking, rather than trying to control outcomes by manipulating phenomena.

Interpretive social science can be criticised for ignoring fundamental aspects of social life, just as positivist social science can be criticised for imposing comparability on people, ignoring individual differences, and neglecting personal perceptions and meanings. Its focus on subjective meaning and communications leaves out of consideration the structural features of social life which constrain choice and strongly influence how people think and live. When structural factors beyond an individual's control, such as poverty, racial and gender stereotypes, and unemployment, have such a profound influence it is dishonest to promote improved communications, mutual understanding, and personal change as ways of improving life. This is a form of manipulation and control by science in no less a way than the kind of control which results from a positivist approach.

Both positivist and interpretive social science, then, can become ideologies. An ideology, as defined by Larrain (1979), is a set of ideas which are used by a social class to misrepresent the nature of reality in its own interests and thereby control and manipulate another class, and prevent them from understanding how society really functions. Science—of whatever kind—has become the modern ideology, replacing to some extent religious ideas which were the former ideological controlling ideas.

This view of science as ideology can be applied to nursing models, and it helps us to see why so much attention has been given to them in recent decades. Science, with its focus on rationality, has become the dominant ideology in wider society and nursing, as part of that society, has followed the same path. And because 'real' or positivist science has greater status than interpretive or 'soft' science in society as a whole, so it has become more influential within nursing.

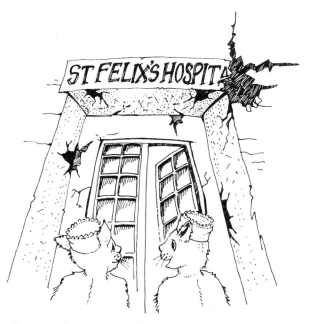

'Structural constraints'?—the structure's falling down, nurse Kitt!

'Real' nursing science?

'Real', positivist science has predominant social status, although this situation may be changing, with wider acknowledgement of the problems surrounding positivist methods and the inevitable influence of personal values on all kinds of research. Nevertheless, within nursing positivism is still the favoured approach and therefore nursing is 'about a decade behind the times' (Silva & Rothbart 1984:8).

Nursing models derived from systems theory are in the positivist tradition, as evidenced by Putt (1978), who states that a nurse using systems theory 'must decide whether to support, to contract or to stabilise the forces at work' (p34) upon the patient. The nurse-scientist 'must identify her goal' (p34) and 'the patient can be guided towards a more objective view of his (sic) disease process' (p167). Thus, the objective nurse understands the situation of the patient without reference to her/his perceptions of the situation, which are not 'objective'. Systems theory, like behaviourist psychology, is not concerned with people's perceptions or interpretations of their own situations, and therefore appropriate methods of nursing intervention or 'manipulation' are 'learning by reinforcement' and 'consistency of feedback' (Putt 1978:13). This mechanistic view of human beings denies their very humanity and treats them like computers which receive input, process it automatically and without thinking, and produce output (Ellis 1982, Kasch 1984). The same concepts are evident in the idea of coping or adapting 'mechanisms', which suggest an automatic process, devoid of thought and emotion.

Roy's adaptation model of nursing (Riehl & Roy 1980) is an example of a systems-based and therefore positivist model. Roy starts off by identifying a human being as a whole entity, a biopsychosocial being, but then fragments this being into four modes, or subsystems, namely the physiological, self-concept, interdependence and role-function modes. Adaptation is said to take place in these four modes in response to stimuli which may be focal (an immediate stimulus or stressor), contextual (present in the environment at that time), or residual (an influence from the past). The role of the nurse is to promote adaptation in a maladapting or sick person by manipulating these stimuli. Thus, it is the nurse who decides what constitutes adaptation and desirable patient outcomes and, by manipulating stimuli which may be the patient's behaviours, beliefs and attitudes, she is in reality manipulating the patient her/himself. How this 'man-ipulation' is to be achieved and how adaptation and maladaption are defined are not considered by Roy. In an example of the application of her model to a sick child and an anxious mother, she makes no reference to validating nursing judgements with clients, and identifies a successful outcome as 'the patient is functioning adequately in the modified parenting role' which the nurse 'prescribes' (Chaska 1983:462).

Orem's self-care model (1980) is another systems-influenced, positivist-type model, according to Orem herself and to Riehl and Roy (1980). Although Orem uses the term 'nursing system', this is not developed along the lines of general systems theory, and her model may perhaps be better classified as 'developmental' (Fawcett 1984). Developmental approaches, however, do not escape the criticism of being mechanistic and positivist because they view all humans as moving along the same line of development, whether this is towards self-care (Orem 1980), maturity (Peplau: see Riehl & Roy 1980), or self-actualisation (Maslow: see Riehl & Roy 1980). Like Roy, Orem places the nurse-scientist in the pre-eminent position, for it is s/he who 'designs nursing systems' for individual patients. In a similar way to Roy, she also begins from a holistic definition of an individual but

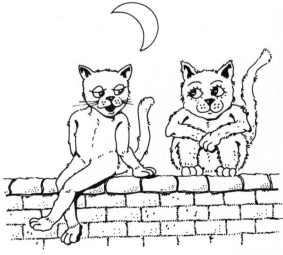

You can manipulate my focal stimuli any time you like sweetie!

reduces her/him later to a set of 'self-care needs' (Meleis 1985:173).

The sociology of knowledge is the study of how ideas emerge and become established as part of social life as a whole, and not as an isolated event. Fundamental to this approach is the notion that ideas cannot become accepted and widespread unless they fit in with other commonly-held ideas. If Orem's self-care theory, which was developed in the USA, is considered in this way we can see that her ideas fit very well with a private insurance-based health care system. Patients are under pressure to be discharged from hospital or the care of their doctor and to become self-caring as soon as possible, because their insurance may not cover them for all the expenses they incur in a longer treatment or for certain kinds of non-technical (i.e. basic nursing) care. Therefore, Orem's model is appropriate to such a system of health care because it defines a successful outcome as a return to self-care as soon as possible (Melnyck 1983). Such a model may not be appropriate to a

National Health Service as we have traditionally known it, with its preventive care emphasis and its provision of care without direct payment at the time of use. However, it is not difficult to envisage a time when, with increasing privatisation of the National Health Service, Orem's model might also fit well in the UK. Indeed it is even possible to anticipate how the adoption of a model like Orem's might actually help to pave the way for fundamental changes in the provision of health care in the UK by forming part of a process of promoting self-care and early return to 'community care'. There is not space here for a full discussion of the implications of community care policies which, because they are based on notions of cost-cutting rather than quality of care, are in fact ways of passing the responsibility for care over to individuals—and especially women, who are defined as society's carers (Finch & Groves 1984, Webb 1985). But it is easy to see how nursing models based on concepts of self-care and individual rather than social responsibility might be used for wider political purposes, and this is another reason why nurses need to be fully conscious of the hidden assumptions of the models they may use in their everyday practice. A fully-fledged profession is one which faces up to its social responsibilities, and does not blindly implement what others propose (Hardy 1982).

Both the Roy and Orem approaches, then, focus on individuals and their problems, and underemphasise environmental or social influences, in the way that many others do. This relatively asociological approach is exemplified in the fact that Stevens (1979) does not even include society or the environment as a concept to be examined when evaluating nursing models (Flaskerud & Halloran 1980). Furthermore, the individual is broken down into a set of sub-systems, nursing is reduced to a set of functions, and the illness-problem-maladaptation emphasis of the medical model is much in evidence (Meleis 1985). The individuality and subjectivity of nurse and patient/client are not part of the agenda in this type of model, or they are grafted on in an attempt to humanise what is a fundamentally a human philosophical approach.

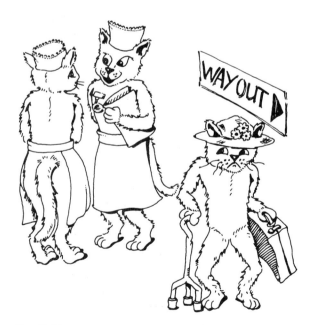

Our Self-care model soon gets them standing on their own two feet!

'Soft' nursing science?

Interactionist and existential nursing models fall into the category of interpretive or 'soft' science, and King's model is one of these. This type of model focusses on the nurse–patient relationship and sees nursing goals as being achieved through a process of working together to arrive at shared perceptions of a situation, setting mutually-agreed goals, and achieving these largely by communications and counselling techniques. Thus, the individual patient is treated as a unique person with particular beliefs, attitudes and definitions of the situation, and nursing care focusses on this individual.

The world beyond this interpersonal relationship is put 'in brackets', and the structural constraints and influences on health are thereby ignored. Diseases of poverty, or the depression of an isolated housewife or someone in an alienating, conveyor-belt job cannot be cured through communications and improved nurse–patient interactions. All that can be hoped for is that the patient will adjust to the situation, conform to social norms, and not disrupt the system by deviant or illness behaviour.

A further complication not considered in interactionist models is that communications and interaction are themselves subject to structural constraints (Kasch 1984). The nurse–patient relationship is one of unequal power because the nurse is a professional to whom the patient comes for help with a problem, and this inequality will affect communications no matter how open and accepting the nurse tries to be. Another constraint may well be differences in educational levels and articulateness in communications between nurse and patient, which weights the scales against equality (Kasch 1984). In stating that human beings 'can transcend the given situation' (Ellis 1982: 352) and that they are 'free agent(s) and free to set (their) own goals' (Ellis 1982: 354), these theorists are therefore engaging in an ideological deception and implying that all problems have their origins and solutions within the individual.

King's work can also be criticised for focussing to a much greater extent on the patient's side of the nursing relationship, and giving relatively little consideration to the perceptions, needs and interaction of the nurse.

Coming together?

A combination of approaches is used by Henderson (1958) and by Roper, Logan and Tierney (1980), whose Activities of Living (AL) model is derived from Henderson's work. Aggleton and Chalmers (1985) detect elements of both a positivist, behaviourist influence and interactionism. Roper's model is reductionist, in reducing a person originally conceptualised as a holistic being to 12 Activities of Living. The biopsychosocial definition of the human being is also unevenly applied, with relatively greater emphasis on the biological, less on the psychological, and least on the sociological aspects.

Roy has recently tried to meet criticism of her adaptation model by incorporating an emphasis on the importance of patients' or clients' definitions of the situation, and agreeing goals and interventions with them (Roy & Roberts 1981). However, this leads to an internal inconsistency between two approaches, as Kasch points out when he asks:

> how nurses should reconcile the demands for authenticity in relationships with the 'responsibility to control and manipulate environmental variables to restore a steady state'.
>
> (Kasch 1984:75)

He goes on to observe that

> because systems theory had little to say about the underlying process of communication, it is never clear how communication might be used strategically in the intervention phase of the nursing process. . . . systems thinking has not contributed much to understanding caregiver–patient interaction in the delivery of nursing care.
>
> (Kasch 1984:75)

King introduces the terminology of systems theory into the explanation of her model, thereby running the risk of philosophical incompatibility with her interactionist approach. However, the systems aspect is given relatively little emphasis and Fawcett (1984) does not consider that the model is undermined by this. This comment applies equally to Roper's attempt to fuse two contradictory philosophical approaches.

Another possible contradiction for 'soft' models lies in their adoption of the nursing process as the vehicle for implementation of their ideas. The nursing process is simply a problem-solving approach and is very similar to 'the scientific method', with its positivist associations with notions of controlling people. Is there a fundamental incompatibility, then, in combining the nursing process with an interactionist, 'soft' model? This difficulty may perhaps be overcome by insisting on a joint approach to all stages of the nursing process by both nurse and patient or client. King's model involves mutual goal-setting, and this has in fact been shown to lead to improved goal achievement (See O'Neill, Chapter 5 of this book). Mutual agreement would have to be extended to all stages of the nursing process in order to eliminate contradictions with an interpretive nursing model, but how far this is feasible is open to doubt because, although patients or clients could conceivably validate their nursing assessment and actual problems, they may have difficulty with some potential problems and nursing interventions due to lack of knowledge and no realistic possibility of making an informed choice.

In summary, the shared features of different types of models lie in their focus on the isolated individual and neglect of social influences on health, ill-health and health care, which amounts to a 'take care of yourself' or 'victim-blaming' position. All models considered here take off from a holistic stance but go on to reduce people to lists of needs, activities or modes of adapting, and thereby fragment the concept of biopsycho-social unity. All the models also have ideological connotations and political consequences, because of their suggestions about manipulating people and their beliefs, either by ignoring their own perceptions and subjectivity or by implying that all problems can be solved by improved inter-personal relationships. As such, they all make the nurse into an agent of social control and, as

Palisin (1971) has said of the nursing process, are 'a snare and a delusion' for nurse and patient alike.

So where do we go from here?

Fay (1975) has identified a third approach which is a development beyond both positivist and interpretive science. This third persepective is that of the critical theorist who seeks, not to control people through prediction or interpersonal relationships, but to study social life in order to help people to change those aspects which they would like to change. This is done by using the critical method of integrating theory and practice, in which social theory plays an educative role. The theorist-practitioner seeks to raise people's consciousness by helping them to analyse and understand their own situations, and by showing them alternative ways of viewing these situations and the factors which influence their lives for good or ill. The goal of critical theory is the enlightenment of social actors themselves and not the social scientist, as in the positivist and interpretive versions. In this way, actors participate in research, or in our case in their own care planning, and 'actively engage in deciding what it is they are and want, and what arrangements must be altered or established to fulfil themselves' (Fay 1975:105). Naturally the critical theorist-practitioner must be prepared for occasions when people reject the new ideas s/he is trying to introduce, and it would be incompatible with the philosophy of the critical approach to impose anything upon them. This educative process also involves interaction between the critical theorist-nurse and patients or clients, so that nurses also come to re-assess who they are, what they want, and the social conditions in which they work. Critical theory therefore involves a dialectic or two-way trans-action between theory and practice, and between nurse and patient or client. It allows nurses to change their role from that of 'doctor's advocate' to 'patient's advocate' (Ashley 1980), by seeing the world from the patient's or client's side and not from the medical perspective, as they do by default when using the nursing process without a nursing philosophical background.

The chapters which follow catalogue nurses' attempts to criticise, modify and use a nursing approach. Readers will be able to consider the model-based care plans in each chapter in the light of the questions already raised about the kinds of theoretical thinking they embody. They will also be able to consider whether these approaches and the values they represent are compatible with their own beliefs about nursing, and they will begin to form a judgement about the theory–models–conceptual framework debate discussed at the beginning of this introductory chapter. In the postscript, the conclusions of individual chapter authors will be brought together, and an evaluation will be made of the intellectual and scientific status of the nursing models used, and of their appropriateness to the British nursing context.

References

Aggleton P & Chalmers H 1985 6. Roper's activities of living model. *Nursing Times*, 13 February: 59–61

American Nurses' Association 1980 *Nursing. A social policy statement.* American Nurses' Association, Kansas

Ashley JA 1980 Power in structured misogyny: implications for the politics of care. *Advances in Nursing Science*, **2**, 3:3–22

Chaska NL (ed) 1983 *The nursing profession. A time to speak.* McGraw-Hill, New York

Cicourel A 1964 *Method and measurement in sociology.* Free Press, New York

Dickoff J, James P & Weidenbach E 1968 Theory in a practice discipline. *Nursing Research*, **17**, 5:415–435

Ellis R 1982 Conceptual issues in nursing. *Nursing Outlook*, July-August: 406–410

Fawcett J 1984 *Analysis and evaluation of conceptual models of nursing.* FA Davis, Philadelphia

Fay B 1975 *Social theory and political practice.* George Allen & Unwin, London

Finch J & Groves D 1983 *A labour of love. Women, work and caring.* Routledge & Kegan Paul, London

Flaskerud JH & Halloran EJ 1980 Areas of agreement in nursing theory development. *Advances in Nursing Science*, **3**, 1:1–7

Fowler HW & Fowler FG 1973 *Concise Oxford Dictionary.* Oxford University Press, Oxford

Freidson E 1977 The future of professionalisation. In: Stacey M, Reid M, Heath C & Dingwall R (Eds) *Health and the division of labour.* Croom Helm, London

Glaser BG & Strauss AL 1967 *The discovery of grounded theory: strategies for qualitative research.* Aldine Press, Chicago

Goode WJ & Hatt PK 1952 *Methods in social research.* McGraw-Hill, New York

Gordon M 1982 *Nursing diagnosis. Process and application.* McGraw-Hill, New York

Hardy L 1982 Nursing models and research—a restricting view? *Journal of Advanced Nursing*, 7:447–451

Henderson V 1958 *Basic principles of nursing care.* International Council of Nurses, London

Huff D 1979 *How to lie with statistics.* Penguin, Harmondsworth

Johnson DE 1959 The nature of a science of nursing. *Nursing Outlook*, 7:291–294

Kasch C 1984 Interpersonal competence and communication in the delivery of nursing care. *Advances in Nursing Science*, **6**, 2:71–88

Lancaster W & Lancaster J 1981 Models and model building in nursing. *Advances in Nursing Science*, **3**, 3:31–42

Larrain J 1979 *The concept of ideology.* Hutchinson, London

Mannheim K 1966 *Ideology and utopia.* Routledge & Kegan Paul, London

Meleis AI 1985 *Theoretical nursing. Development and progress.* JB Lippincott, Philadelphia

Melnyck KAM 1983 The process of theory analysis: an examination of the nursing theory of Dorothea E Orem. *Nursing Research*, **32**, 3:170–174

Menke EM   1983   Critical analysis of theory development in nursing. In: Chaska NL (Ed) *The nursing profession: a time to speak.* McGraw-Hill, New York

National League for Nursing 1983 *Criteria for the evaluation of baccalaureate and higher degree programs in nursing.* National League for Nursing, New York

Orem DE   1980   *Nursing: concepts of practice* (2nd edition) McGraw-Hill, New York

Palisin HE   1971   Nursing care plans are a snare and a delusion. *American Journal of Nursing*, January: 63–66

Putt AM   1978   *General systems theory applied to nursing.* Little, Brown, Boston

Rambo BJ   1984   *Adaptation nursing. Assessment and intervention.* WB Saunders, Philadelphia

Riehl JP & Roy C   1980   *Conceptual models for nursing practice.* Appleton-Century-Crofts, New York

Rogers M   1963   Some comments on the theoretical basis for nursing practice. *Nursing Science*, **63**, 1:11–13, 60–61

Roper N, Logan WW & Tierney AJ   1980   *The elements of nursing.* Churchill Livingstone, Edinburgh

Roy C   1983   Theory development in nursing: proposal for direction. In: Chaska NL (Ed) *The nursing profession: a time to speak.* McGraw-Hill, New York

Roy C & Roberts S   1981   *Theory construction in nursing: an adaptation model.* Prentice-Hall, New Jersey

Silva MC & Rothbart D   1984   An analysis of changing trends in philosophies of science on nursing theory development and testing (sic). *Advances in Nursing Science*, **6**, 2:1–13

Spender D   1981   The gatekeepers: a feminist critique of academic publishing. In: Roberts H (Ed) *Doing Feminist Research.* Routledge & Kegan Paul, London

Stevens BJ   1979   *Nursing theory. Analysis, application, evaluation.* Little, Brown, Boston

Thibodeau JA   1983   *Nursing models: analysis and evaluation.* Wadsworth, California

Walker LO   1983   Theory and research in the development of nursing as a discipline: retrospect and prospect. In Chaska NL (Ed) *The nursing profession: a time to speak.* McGraw-Hill, New York

Webb C   1984a   On the eighth day god created the nursing process—and nobody rested. *Senior Nurse*, **1**, 33:22–25

Webb C   1984b   A nursing study of recovery from hysterectomy. Unpublished PhD thesis, University of London

Webb C   1985   *Sexuality, nursing and Health.* J Wiley, Chichester

Williams CA   1979   The nature and development of conceptual frameworks. In Downs FS & Fleming JW (Eds) *Issues in nursing research.* Appleton-Century-Crofts, New York

Wright Mills C   1959   *The sociological imagination.* Oxford University Press, London

2

Care plan for a woman having ante-natal care, based on Orem's Self-care model

Rosemary Methven

This Chapter was undertaken as part of an MSc course in Nursing at Manchester University. A descriptive study of the ante-natal booking interview was undertaken on forty women, evenly distributed at four maternity hospitals. During their booking clinic visit these women were also interviewed by the researcher-author using a nursing process semi-structured interview schedule based on the Self-care Model of Orem (1980). This had the main objective of assessing how much data relevant to the woman's care during pregnancy had not been ascertained during the initial booking interview.

The following study has been chosen at random to demonstrate the relevance of Orem's Self-care Model to maternity care and to illustrate the quantity and quality of relevant information on which midwifery care can be based in comparison to that recorded on the ante-natal frontsheet (obstetric record). The care-plan is hypothetical because the nature of the overall research study did not allow follow-up care of the mothers interviewed but served to demonstrate how the material obtained at interview could be used for future care in line with Orem's model.

The concept of Self-care

> Self-care is the practice of activities that individuals initiate and perform on their own behalf in maintaining life, health and well-being.
> (Orem 1980:35)

Orem (1980) gives the above definition of self-care, explaining that 'self' is used in the sense of one's 'whole being'. Self-care, she maintains, is the requirement of every person, and when it is

not performed, 'illness, disease or death will occur'. In other words, where people are caring for themselves holistically, in terms of their physical, psychological, emotional and spiritual make-up and social environment, a condition of health should be obtained. 'Health' here is viewed according to the World Health Organisation (1947) definition, as

> A state of complete physical, mental and social well-being, and not merely the absence of disease or infirmity.

Orem believes that nursing is required only when the adult is unable to continuously maintain the amount or quality of self-care which is therapeutic in sustaining life and health, recovery from disease and injury, or recovery from their effects. In the case of children, she maintains that the nursing function is justified when the parents or guardians are 'unable to continuously maintain for the child, the amount or quality of care that is therapeutic'. This is particularly apposite to the role of the midwife.

Reasons for failure of a person's normal self-care practice are many and varied. Physical disorder or disease for example may temporarily or permanently render a person incapable of performing certain necessary functions, such as eating. Mental disease or emotional disorder may affect a person's desire to eat, even though the person is physically capable of eating. Social or environmental conditions may make eating difficult or impossible, despite the physical ability and desire to eat. Religious practice may dictate how or what is eaten, which in some circumstances may be detrimental to physical health. Lack of knowledge may prevent people eating that which is good for health and sometimes may even allow them to eat that which is harmful, thereby promoting disease. Any of these situations may contribute to a breakdown in self-care and so render the person in need of nursing care.

The concept of nursing

Nursing function must be viewed in relation to the philosophy of nursing held by that person (Stevens 1979). In common with Henderson (1966), who regards nursing as 'assisting the person, sick or well, in the performance of those activities . . . which he would normally perform unaided, if he had the necessary strength, will or knowledge', Orem views nursing as 'action which enables the patient to accomplish self-care' and 'action to compensate for, or to overcome the person's inability, or limited ability to engage in self-care'.

Nursing is viewed by both these authors as a compensatory function, the nurse supplying whatever action the patient needs in terms of knowledge, will or strength to perform usual activities or engage in those behaviours related to treatment prescribed by the physician. Nursing is thus a 'helping art' (Hinchcliff 1979) and, as such, is consistent with the concept of the midwife as one who 'helps' the mother (Myles 1975).

Orem states that there are at least five general methods which one person, in the capacity of nurse, can use to give help or assistance to another. They are:

1   Acting or doing for another
2   Guiding another
3   Supporting another (physically or psychologically)
4   Providing an environment that promotes personal development in relation to becoming able to meet present or future demands for action
5   Teaching another

These methods, Orem states, are applicable in a variety of situations, namely in a hospital, community or within the family. They also depend on the status of the patient. Thus, for people who are unable to engage in any form of deliberate action, for example if they anaesthetised or in a coma, the nurse's care will be totally compensatory. If the people have mental faculties, and are able to make decisions or judgements about their care but lack the physical ability to carry them out, the nurse's role is partly compensatory. Similarly, a person may be unable to make rational decisions about therapeutic self-care, perhaps because of lack of knowledge, but if helped to understand what is required, may be able to perform it effectively. In this instance the nurse would be exercising a 'supportive/educative' role.

The concept of midwifery

Little has been written about the role of the midwife from a philosophical point of view (Robinson, Golden & Bradley 1981) though the definition of 'being with the woman in order to help' the mother (Myles 1975) is everywhere implicit. Walker (1976) identifies 'three basic elements of the midwifery ideology' as 'the concept of normality, the idea of continuity of care and the responsibility of the midwife as a practitioner in her own right'. Walker also contends that, because many midwives have had previous training as a nurse, they are more likely to accept an 'illness model' of childbirth and continue to behave as nurses while working within the obstetric field. She also feels that working within the hospital context and administrative structure is likely to strengthen the 'nursing rather than the midwifery behaviour'. The same point is made by Donnison (1979). She writes

> Midwives . . . are traditionally trained as nurses before becoming midwives. They may thus come into midwifery conditioned by their authoritarian, hospital-based nurse training, to regard the childbearing woman as 'sick' and to accept too readily the prevailing medical view of what is in her interest.

Donnison also notes the importance of continuity

of care for the mother and adds that it is from this that 'midwives derive their main job satisfaction'. She states that

> Many midwives argue that, with careful organis-
> ation, it *is* possible to ensure that the woman has
> continuity of care by a person or persons already
> known to her.

The analysis of the nurse's role, delineated by Orem, would appear to be wholly consistent with the concept of the midwife being 'with the mother' in order to 'help' her during a normal pregnancy, delivery and puerperium. In this way the status of the mother is not reduced to that of 'patient' and the ideal of a 'partnership of care' remains possible, by a single midwife or team of midwives (Thomson 1980). The midwife will give partly compensatory care to the woman during labour and in some instances during a complicated pregnancy or puerperium.

On the rare occasion when a woman does require a general anaesthetic or is comatosed due to eclampsia, the midwife's care becomes 'totally compensatory'. She also cares for neonates if they are rejected by their mothers or, where the mother for some reason is unable to provide the necessary care, the midwife will give totally or partly compensatory care to the baby.

Generally, however, the midwife's care for the mother during the ante-natal and post-natal periods should be 'supportive/educative', because the mother should be encouraged to perform her own self-care and give 'dependent self-care' to her baby.

Elements of Orem's nursing model

Orem identified three types of self-care requisites. They are defined as follows:

1 *Universal self-care requisites.* These are common to all human beings during all stages of the life cycle, and are adjusted according to age, developmental state, environment and other factors.
2 *Developmental self-care requisites.* These are associated with human developmental processes and conditions and events during various stages of the life cycle, e.g. prematurity and pregnancy.
3 *Health deviation self-care requisites.* These are associated with genetic and constitutional defects and human structural–functional deviation, together with their effects, medical diagnosis and treatment.

Orem's theory of nursing relates readily to the philosophy of midwifery. Developmental requisites relate specifically to the developing fetus and neonate as well as to those changes accompanying pregnancy, labour and the puerperium for the mother. Health deviation self-care requisites relate to the complications when the nurse or midwife 'seeks and participates in medical care for health deviations and self-care actions'. The eight Universal Health Care Requisites relate to a person's pattern of everyday living and maintenance of normal health. They are

1 The maintenance of a sufficient intake of air.
2 The maintenance of a sufficient intake of water.
3 The maintenance of a sufficient intake of food.
4 The provision of care associated with elimination processes and excretion.
5 The maintenance of a balance between rest and activity.
6 The maintenance of a balance between solitude and social interaction.
7 The prevention of hazard to human life, human functioning and human well-being.
8 The promotion of human functioning and development within social groups in accord with human potential, known human limitations, and the human desire to be normal. Normalcy is used in the sense of that which is essentially human, and that which is in accord with the genetic and constitutional characteristics and the talents of individuals.

(Orem 1980)

The Department of Health and Social Security (1977) in the series on *Prevention and Health, Reducing the Risk, Safer Pregnancy and Childbirth*, states

> The individual and the family can do much to help themselves and others by assuming greater personal responsibility for their own health and well-being.

Orem's eight universal self-care requisites were felt to be appropriate for any pregnant mother and to provide a suitable base line from which both the physical and psychological effects of pregnancy on a woman could be measured. Developmental self-care requisites were felt to have been adequately covered by the conventional ante-natal booking interview. It was decided not to duplicate this information, and therefore developmental self-care requisites were disregarded. Health deviation self-care requisites were considered to be irrelevant for the purpose of the present study, which concentrates on a woman who expects to be in a state of normal health.

The need for a framework

> A theoretical framework is imperative as a basis for nursing practice.

This statement by Venables (1980) typifies a stance taken by other authors, including Schlotdfelt (1975), Reilly (1975), Stevens (1979) and McFarlane (1980). Dickoff and James (1968) maintain that a theory for a professional or practice discipline (such as nursing or midwifery) must go beyond description and prediction and must provide a conceptualisation specifically intended to guide the shaping of reality to that profession's professional purpose. This would suggest that a model should be designed specifically for midwifery and use by midwives.

A unique midwifery model may well be necessary and may come to fruition in the future, but none exists at present. It is therefore necessary to utilise a model that has already been tried, even though it was originally designed for use in general nursing. In selecting a model on which to base a nursing process assessment for use in the present study, the following considerations were identified as relevant and important:

1 Pregnancy and childbirth are judged to be states of normal, if altered health and not conditions of illness. (McKinlay 1972, Oakley 1979)

2 Midwifery care should aim to support the mother in her own health care and not to encourage dependency on the midwife.

3 The new-born baby is totally dependent, and the mother's/parents' normal role is therefore to provide total care for this infant.

4 The midwife's role is to support the parents by providing education and supervision as necessary, giving only such assistance as may be required until the mother/parents are competent enough to care for the child independently.

5 The province of the midwife is the care of both mother and baby provided that their health and progress remain within normal limits.

6 Any abnormality or deviation from normal in either mother or baby requires the midwife to refer to the obstetrician or paediatrician. Subsequently, her role is to continue to provide such care as is needed and to follow the doctor's instructions.

7 The midwife's role involves practical skills, education and counselling in preventive health, and the ability to develop a relationship of trust with the mother and the health care team. These involve communications and interpersonal skills.

8 Mothers and parents today are frequently well-informed about pregnancy and childbirth and often hold widely differing views about the conduct of delivery and method of childbearing. The midwife's role is to support the parents and not to impose her own views, providing there is no risk involved to either mother or baby.

Choosing an appropriate model

A model based on interpersonal or interactive skills, such as those proposed by King (1975) (see Chapter 5) or Riehl (1980), might be appropriate for use in midwifery. Sundeen *et al.* (1976) demonstrate the use of an interaction model for the care of the ante-natal woman. However, while care during pregnancy, labour and the puerperium most definitely depends on the establishment of an effective relationship based on mutual interpersonal skills and communication, this is inappropriate when applied to the neonate. It is essential that the model applies equally well to both mother and baby, and therefore interaction models were discarded.

Roy's Adaptation Model (1976) (see Chapter 8) seemed appropriate for several reasons. It complied with the criteria set out by Riehl and Roy (1980) as a design that provides the most complete view of the person with the least number of categories, which they term parsimony. It is appropriate to the pregnant woman, in that she undergoes marked physiological changes in every bodily system. Her self-concept and role function may change with the onset of pregnancy and motherhood, while her interdependence and relationships are vitally important in this context.

Downey (1980) demonstrated the use of the Roy Adaptation Model with a maternity patient with some success. However, the analysis is not appropriate for the neonate. In addition it was felt that midwives in this country currently do not generally have a sufficient knowledge base to cope with the underlying theory of psychology and adaptation. This means that while it might be possible to make an assessment of the pregnant woman using the Roy Adaptation Model, design of the care plan in order to manipulate the focal, contextual and residual stimuli (Roy 1976) would be more difficult.

Another disadvantage with this model is its negative connotation when the health state of the mother and baby are considered to be essentially normal. This is because deviations from normal, in whatever mode they occur, are listed as problems. Therefore this model was also rejected for the purpose of the present study.

In view of these factors, it was felt that the model of nursing proposed by Orem (1958) and revised in 1980 was most applicable to midwifery practice in Great Britain. It was considered sufficiently straightforward to be comprehended by the majority of midwives, who do not have a background in psychology or sociology, and it does not relegate the healthy mother and her baby to the status of patients. Moreover, its concepts apply equally well to the independent woman in pregnancy as to the dependent neonate at birth.

The underlying philosophy of self-care on which Orem's model is based allows the woman to participate in her own ante-natal and post-natal care. In addition, although this model does utilise a problem-solving approach to care, it does not delineate patient-problems. Instead, the terms 'Health Care Requisites' and 'Health Care Deficits' are used, overcoming the negative connotation conveyed by other terminology.

Because the model was being used to assess women who are essentially well, the order of Orem's universal self-care requisites was altered. This was in line with Moser and Kalton's (1971) recommendation that interview schedules should commence with easily answered, straightforward questions and progress to more sensitive topics when the confidence of the respondent has been obtained.

Orem described the general sets of actions for meeting the eight self-care requisites and the assessment questions were phrased after consideration of her guidelines. They include questions designed to measure the mother's behaviour and habits before and during the present pregnancy as well as an assessment of her present knowledge about health in general and in pregnancy, labour and the post-natal period. From this knowledge it was hoped to be able to construct a care plan with the mother to meet her physical, educational and psychological needs.

Construction of an antenatal assessment schedule based on Orem's Self-care model

An assessment schedule was devised based on Orem's model and this is shown in Figure 2.1. Questions were arranged in sections according to the model; for ethical and humanitarian reasons these were designed to avoid duplication of questions likely to have been asked during the conventional hospital booking history.

A structured assessment schedule with the same questions asked of each mother was used to ensure that all the desired information was covered and data was collected systematically from them all. However, the questions were not always asked in the same order, and some were developed by further probing questions if this appeared desirable to the flow of the conversation or the collection of vital facts.

Open questions were used whenever possible to allow women from different cultures and backgrounds to answer in ways appropriate to them. During the pilot study, however, some of the questions were changed from direct or closed to open questions because the answers given anticipated that type of question. In some instances, for example 'Do you know how to care for your teeth in pregnancy?' was asked in preference to the more correct form 'How should you care for your teeth in pregnancy?' because it was less threatening to the mother who was unsure. Her non-verbal cues usually revealed whether she did know about dental care or if she needed to be taught. It was then possible to follow up the 'Do you know. . . ?' closed question with 'How are you going to care for your teeth. . . ?' for more confident women or to give less sure women the information directly. In this way it was possible to make the booking interview not just an information-receiving time for the midwife but an information-giving opportunity as well.

These questions were asked in the booking

Fig. 2.1 Schedule for structured interview based on Orem's self-care framework, used following a conventional booking interview

HOSPITAL. . . . . **DATE**. . . . . **TIME**. . . . . **INTERVIEW CODE**. . . . . . .

I would like to ask you some further questions on topics which are not usually asked when your history is taken. Because I am not working at the hospital, I am not able to give you information which you may not already know, about the topics we talk about. You should ask the hospital midwives to give you this. I would also like to write down all that you say, so I hope you will not find this disturbing. The more you can tell me, the more helpful it will be. Thank you.

Maintenance of a sufficient Intake of Food.

Please would you describe your usual diet in any normal day before you became pregnant.

1a. What would you have for breakfast?

1b. What would you eat at lunchtime?

1c. What would a normal evening meal consist of?

1d. What other snacks might be taken during the day?

1e. Has there been any alteration in your usual eating pattern since you became pregnant?

Fig. 2.1 (continued)

1f.   Do you know what food requirements are recommended during pregnancy?

1g.   Is there anything that we should know about your diet or eating habits for when you are in hospital?

Maintenance of a Sufficient Intake of Water.
2a.   How much fluid would you usually drink in a twenty-four hour period before you became pregnant (in cups)?

2b.   How much milk did you usually have each day (to include that in custard or as yogurt)?

2c.   How much of your total fluid consumption in any day is alcohol?

2d.   Has there been any alteration in your fluid intake or drinking pattern since the start of pregnancy?

2e.   Do you know what fluid requirements are recommended when you are pregnant?

Maintenance of a Balance between Rest and Activity.
3a.   Will you describe your usual pattern of daily activity (how you spend a normal day).

3b.   Does your job require you to stand for long periods or to be on your feet for any length of time?

3c.   Do you pursue any sports or undertake any vigorous exercise?

3d.   Have you made any changes in your activities since pregnancy began?

3e.   How many hours sleep do you usually have each night?

3f.   Has your sleep pattern changed at all since you have been pregnant?

3g.   Do you know what rest and exercise are recommended during pregnancy?

Maintenance of a Sufficient Intake of Air
4a.   Do you usually have any difficulty with breathing or experience any periods of fainting or breathlessness?

4b.   Do you know how breathing may be affected during pregnancy?

Fig. 2.1 (continued)

Provision of Care Associated with Elimination Processes and Excretion.
5a.   Do you usually have your bowels opened every day?

5b.   Are you aware of any tendency to constipation or diarrhoea when you are not pregnant?

5c.   How do you usually cope with this?

5d.   Did you have any trouble with haemorrhoids before you became pregnant?

5e.   Have you noticed any change with your bowels or haemorrhoids since pregnancy began?

5f.   Do you usually pass urine without difficulty?

5g.   Did you usually have to get up at night to go to the toilet before you became pregnant?

5h.   Has there been any alteration in this pattern since you have been pregnant?

5i.   Are you aware of any changes that may occur with your bladder or bowel function now that you are pregnant?

The Promotion of Human Functioning and Development, and the Desire to Be Normal.
6a.   How did you feel when you first realised that you were pregnant?

6b.   How do you feel about being pregnant now?

6c.   What have you read or what do you know about having a baby and becoming a mother?

6d.   What do you think about labour and actually giving birth to a baby?

6e.   How well do you think you (and your husband) will manage a new baby?

6f.   What are your views about feeding the baby?

6g.   Do you know how to care for your breasts during pregnancy?

6h.   Do you know about the Parentcraft Classes that are provided in this hospital?

6i.   Do you plan to attend these?

Fig. 2.1 (continued)

7a.   What changes to your present life-style do you think pregnancy and having a baby will make for you (and your husband)?

7b.   How do you feel about this?

7c.   What family or other support do you have to help you?

7d.   Are there any aspects of your religious practice that might be affected when you are in hospital?

The Prevention of Hazard to Human Life, Functioning and Interaction.

8a.   Do you know what footwear and clothing are recommended while you are pregnant?

8b.   Do you know how to care for your teeth and gums during pregnancy?

8c.   When did you last attend a dentist, or when is your next dental appointment?

8d.   Do you know what things or situations you should avoid during pregnancy because they might be harmful to you and/or your baby?

8e.   Have you taken any steps to avoid these things since pregnancy began?

8f.   What things would make you contact your doctor or the hospital while you are pregnant?

8g.   Is there anything that usually makes you feel stressed or anxious?

8h.   Is there anything about having a baby or being a parent might do to cause you to feel stressed, anxious or embarrassed for example?

Maintenance of a Balance between Solitude and Rest.

9a.   Would you say that you are the sort of person who likes a lot of people around you or do you prefer your own company?

9b.   Have you ever been in hospital before as a patient?

9c.   Have you ever been apart from your husband/children/family before?

9d.   How do you usually react to being apart from your husband/children/family?

9e.   How do they usually react to being apart from you?

Fig. 2.1 (continued)

9f.   How do you think you will cope with being in hospital to have the baby, especially during labour?

9g.   How do you think your husband will cope while you are in hospital?

9h.   What is your reaction to being cared for by hospital staff and midwives whom you may not have met before?

9i.   Do you have any views about students doctors or midwives looking after you while you are at clinic or in hospital?

General Questions and Information.
10.   Is there anything you would like to ask me?

11.   Midwives subjective impression of the mother:

11a. General appearance.

11b. Estimate of apparent intelligence.

11c. Personality.

11d. Social or cultural background.

11e. Language or difficulty with speech.

11f. Any hearing loss or physical feature of note.

Thank you very much for your help and for letting me talk to you.

---

clinic while the women were waiting to see the obstetrician after an initial history had been recorded by the clinic midwife.

Maintenance of a sufficient intake of food (Questions 1a to 1g)

Diet is an important factor in pregnancy and often determines the degree of minor disorders experienced by the mother. Although a dietician may be available in some ante-natal clinics to advise about diet in pregnancy, many women do not see her for a variety of reasons. Midwives are taught to give dietary advice to women in pregnancy, and it was felt that advice about normal diet in a normal pregnancy falls within the remit of the midwife. Thus, women need only be referred to a dietician should dietary problems or conditions occur which require specialist dietary advice, e.g. diabetes. Moreover, an awareness of a woman's usual diet when she is not pregnant is useful information on which to base sound midwifery advice should minor disorders with dietary implications develop later in pregnancy. Questions 1a to 1g were intended to provide a baseline from which the woman's dietary habits could be evaluated for the duration of pregnancy, and from which advice relevant to that woman's needs could be given.

The maintenance of a sufficient intake of water (Questions 2a to 2e)

The renal system is greatly affected by pregnancy. Maintenance of a sufficient intake of fluid can prevent the onset of infection and other complications. Questions 2a to 2e were designed to assess the woman's normal fluid intake, so that appropriate advice could be given where it was required. Calcium is a necessary component of diet in pregnancy in order to supply increased fetal demands. Question 2b is designed to assess the woman's usual intake and to provide an opportunity for introducing calcium into the diet by other means if the mother does not like milk. The effect of alcohol on the fetus is now recognised as a major cause of neonatal disorder, and Woolf (1979) and Plant (1983) comment that ante-natal clinics provide a wonderful opportunity to offer education, sustained support and encouragement to women in order to help those who need to modify excessive alcohol consumption.

Maintenance of a balance between activity and rest (Questions 3a to 3g)

These questions were designed to assess the woman's level of rest and activity before pregnancy, in order that appropriate advice concerning exercise suitable for pregnancy and the recommended amount of rest during the antenatal period could be given. Some work situations, e.g. hair-dressing, require the mother to stand for long periods, predisposing to the development of varicosed veins. Knowledge about this could enable a midwife to discuss ways of preventing their development with the woman. Some women in later pregnancy find difficulty in sleeping. Questions 3e and f were designed to form a base line for comparison later in pregnancy should this situation occur. This might provide a more realistic picture for the doctor needing to decide whether a woman requires sleeping tablets.

Maintenance of a sufficient intake of air (Questions 4a and b)

This self-care requirement is usually inappropriate in a normal healthy woman, and its inclusion might convey suggestions of illness to her. However, for the sake of completeness of the model in use, it was retained but placed in the middle of the list and not, as Orem positioned it, at the start. This was in line with Moser and Kalton's (1971) recommendation for questionnaire and interview schedule design that difficult or sensitive topics should be placed later in the schedule. The inclusion of a question about fainting made the topic more relevant to pregnancy.

Provision of care associated with elimination processes (Questions 5c to 5i)

It was decided to include only care of the bladder and bowels under this heading as questions about vaginal bleeding formed part of the conventional booking interview.

The skin is also over-active in pregnancy, and some people develop skin reactions including chloasma and rashes. However, the latter was considered to be outside the bounds of normal and questions relating to care of the skin were not included. Ptyalism is a minor disorder of pregnancy that occurs for a few women. However, excess salivation and discharges from the nasal mucosa were considered to be abnormal and questions regarding them were also excluded.

Promotion of human functioning and development within social groups in accord with human potential, known human limitations, and the human desire to be normal (Questions 6a to 7d)

Orem enlarges on this self-care requisite by commenting that 'normalcy' is used in the sense of that which is essentially human and that which is in accord with genetic and constitutional characteristics and talents of individuals. It was therefore decided to include the more subjective aspects of a woman's reaction to pregnancy and to include the opportunity for some social and religious practice and feelings to be expressed.

The last question in this section was aimed specifically at the large Moslem community in the locality who are known to prefer women doctors and who follow strict patterns of diet and prayer.

Breast-feeding and parentcraft questions were included because it was known that these topics are not always discussed at booking interview.

Prevention of hazard to human life, human functioning and human well-being (Questions 8a to 8h)

Considering the woman as a holistic being, hazards were considered in the physical and psychological realms. The midwife's role as a health educator was borne in mind and the questions were designed to explore the woman's areas of need for education.

Maintenance of a balance between solitude and social interaction (Questions 9a to 9i)

Although the time the woman may expect to spend in hospital for the delivery of her baby is now very short, varying between six hours and seven days on average, some women may need to spend long periods of time on an ante-natal ward if complications develop during pregnancy. It was with these in mind that the questions were

devised so that an appropriate plan of care could be made should admission to hospital occur, and any particular problems or reactions associated with separation could be anticipated and planned for.

The final two questions relating to being cared for in hospital were based on hospital policy. During pregnancy, the woman becomes familiar with the team of staff working in the ante-natal clinic. When she goes into labour, however, a time which for most women brings the greatest stress, the mother has to relate to an entirely different set of midwives in the delivery suite. Some women object to being cared for by student doctors and midwives. Recognising that they have the right to refuse this, most hospitals have a policy that all women should be asked and their personal permission obtained before care is undertaken by non-qualified staff.

Finally an opportunity was presented for the woman to ask questions which the assessment might have aroused in her mind.

Comparison between the conventional booking history and the nursing process assessment

The ante-natal front sheet (Fig. 2.2)

It indicates what information was available about Noeleen at the conclusion of the booking interview. It consists of some factual details about her personal identity, her husband, their address, and general practitioner, which were obtained by the records clerk. The next section was completed by the interviewing midwife.

Menstrual history
This records the uncertainty concerning the woman's dates. The uterine size was estimated to be ten weeks on vaginal examination, which would give an Expected Date of Delivery between the twentieth and twenty-fifth of January. This was more precise than what Noeleen was told by the student midwife during the interview.

Fig. 2.2 Antenatal Record

ANTENATAL RECORD   BOOKED/EMERGENCY

General Practitioner	Age 33 Years Married 4
DR PAYNE	Maiden Name O'GRADY
	Place of Birth EIRE
NEWTOWN HEALTH	Ethnic Group —
CENTRE	N.H.S. No. —
G.P.'s Tel. No.	Patient's Occupation H/W Next of Kin HUSBAND S/A
443 8010	Husband's Occupation MINER Telephone No. 443 1243

NOELEEN BLANK,
3, HIGH STREET,
NEW TOWN

MENSTRUAL HISTORY

L.M.P. (Normal) ? MID APRIL '82   E.D.D. ? JAN '83   Revised E.D.D. ——

Cycle 4-5/28 Regular/Irregular   Date of Quickening ——

Obstetric History

Date	Place	Maturity	Antenatal	Labour Length Complications Method of Delivery	Puerperium	Sex	Birth weight	SB NND	Health now
JAN. '80	M.H.	42/52	—	LSCS. FOR C.P.D.	WOUND INFECTION	♀	7lbs	—	A+W
OCT. '81	M.H.	39/52	—	LSCS. FOR C.P.D.	—	♀	7lb 15½	—	A+W

MEDICAL & SURGICAL HISTORY

IMMUNE TO RUBELLA. NO JAUNDICE OR HEPATITIS.
USUAL CHILDHOOD ILLNESSES

HUSBAND'S SISTER'S CHILD HAS SPINA BIFIDA

FAMILY HISTORY (Diabetes, Dystrophies, Tuberculosis, Congenital abnormalities, Twins, Hypertension, etc.)

SENSITIVITIES (Allergic disease, skin applications, antibiotics, drugs) —

Previous Blood Transfusions NO	Present Treatment (Antibiotics, hormones, etc.) NONE

Present Pregnancy (include haemorrhage, rubella and other infections since conception)

NO BLEEDING, TIREDNESS.

Contraceptive Technique IUCD	Smoking Habit NONE	Rhesus Positive/Negative	W.R. Positive/Negative	Sickling Present/Absent

Special Instructions (Refer Physician, Paediatrician, etc. Investigations, conduct of delivery)

C.S.

Book (Spec. Unit)/G.P. Unit /Not Book/Pending

A.N. CARE

(Total Hosp)/Shared

Date of return visit ....

Early Discharge   Yes/No

Signature ....

(Ring appropriate word) Date ....

CLERK
MIDWIFE
DOCTOR

1083

The notes do not indicate that a more certain date was ever made explicit to Noeleen. It appears that an ultra-sonic scan was not performed at the booking clinic as a further aid to confirming gestation.

Obstetric history
This indicates the dates of Noeleen's two previous confinements but, without calculation, the present ages of her two children are not highlighted. The record does not show that the first caesarean section was undertaken following a seven hour labour, while the second one was elective. There is no indication of the extent of the later wound infection, its effects on the scar, or its method of treatment. However, because the care was given at the same hospital these facts would be available by reference to previous notes.

It is considered that using a symbol to indicate the sex of the children depersonalises them even more than using an abbreviation 'M' or 'F' and that 'A&W' conveys little impression of their present state of health, or the care requirement needed to be given to these children by their mother.

History of present pregnancy
This indicates tiredness which, although a feature of normal pregnancy in the early months, in this case was felt to be exacerbated by depression. The interviewing midwife did not identify this however. Noeleen's other problems are not recorded because they were not discovered.

Medical and surgical history
Several items were identified using Orem's framework that were not specified on the front-sheet, but the note regarding the sister-in-law's child with spina bifida does not tally with the information gained at the assessment interview. It is apparent from the latter that there were two children in the sister-in-law's family with spina bifida, which would suggest a strong genetic tendency (Goodman & Gorlin 1983).

Contraceptive technique
This ante-natal front-sheet demonstrates the separation of this item from the Menstrual History, and indicates how midwives 'starting at the top and working down' the sheet could investigate this topic without relating it to the woman's last menstrual period. 'IUCD' does not specify the type of intrauterine contraceptive device Noeleen was using, nor does it indicate the fact that her pregnancy represents a case of failed contraception. At the time of booking the device was still *in situ*, although the mother did make this clear to the midwife during the interview. A doctor did make a note to this effect in another part of the obstetric record.

Although additional information is available about this woman because of her previous confinements in the same hospital, for a primi-gravida or a woman booking for the first time at this hospital the recorded information would represent the sum total of data available on which to base both her obstetric and midwifery care.

While the notes are clear, easy to follow and concise, they lack the detail with which to make the record and the care personal. Noeleen does not emerge as a person with hopes, fears, personality and opinions. The midwifery aspects of her history are entirely absent; for example, her emotional response to past and present pregnancies and delivery; the method of feeding previously employed and anticipated this time; her present work-load, with two children under two-and-a-half years old to care for and to make arrangements for while she is in hospital for her third caesarean section, and while coming to clinic for ante-natal care. This woman's difficulty with diet and eating is not apparent, although weight gain would be detected at future follow-up visits. However, at best this would be in a month's time, and it could even be six weeks before she visited the clinic again. A great deal of excess weight could be gained in this time and its effect on the pregnancy is incalculable. Its effects on Noeleen's emotional state was not even considered.

This particular booking interview, conducted by a student midwife, lasted just under ten minutes. There was very little additional interaction to that recorded on the front-sheet. Noeleen was not given an opportunity to ask questions, but some brief information was given about the rest of the booking clinic. Further care in pregnancy was not mentioned, and there was no reference to feeding the baby or to parentcraft or relaxation classes.

The nursing process assessment (Fig. 2.3).

In contrast the assessment based on Orem's model does mention pregnancy, and identifies relevant problems that require both midwifery and obstetric intervention.

Noeleen emerges clearly as a person in her own right, with a distinct personality. The quality of her relationship with her husband, other children, wider family and neighbours is apparent. Her life and habits prior to pregnancy indicate the marked change her unplanned pregnancy has brought. Her reaction to this, and to the future caesarean section and sterilisation, are very ob-

vious and provide clues to the type of care and support she may need as term approaches.

The nursing process assessment did take longer than the conventional booking history and it is recognised that the student midwife was inexperienced. However it is considered that, given the opportunity, Noeleen would have 'opened up' and talked about her problems. One reason that the nursing process assessment took longer was because, in the absence of anyone else available to give support, this woman was allowed to talk and weep freely. Because diet was a sensitive issue for her, she was on the verge of tears by the second question and broke down when asked to indicate her pattern of daily activity. It was then that her depression truly emerged, and an apparently innocent question obtained important information without direct probing.

Fig. 2.3 Assessment of Noeleen Blank

Name *Noeleen Blank*.   No. _____   Date 23.6.'82.

Maintenance of a Sufficient Intake of Food

Please would you describe your usual diet in any normal day before you became pregnant.

1a. What would you have for breakfast?
2 slices of bacon, 2 eggs, 1 slice of toast.

1b. What would you eat at lunchtime?
Ryvita with cheese and a tomato

1c. What would a normal evening meal consist of?
Salad and steak with vegetables

1d. What other snacks might be taken during the day?
None

1e. Has there been any alteration in your usual eating pattern since you became pregnant?
"Definitely-that is my problem. I was on a diet before pregnancy & lost 2 stone 9 lbs. I was 11 stone 11 lbs after my last baby born. I never ate carbohydrate before. Now I can't stop eating chocolate & sweet stuff. I've put on 7 lbs in two weeks."

1f. Do you know what food requirements are recommended during pregnancy?
Yes I didn't want to get pregnant. So I'm going to eat now and enjoy myself while I am pregnant. I'm not going to see a dietician.

1g. Is there anything that we should know about your diet or eating habits for when you are in hospital?
No. (looks upset)

Fig. 2.3 (continued)

Maintenance of a Sufficient Intake of Water

2a. **How much fluid would you usually drink in a twenty-four hour period before you became pregnant (in cups)?**
8-mostly cups of tea.

2b. **How much milk did you usually have each day? (to include that in custard or as yogurt)?**
I was allowed $\frac{1}{2}$ pint of milk on my diet and I stuck to that.

2c. **How much of your total fluid consumption in any day is alcohol?**
None.

2d. **Has there been any alteration in your fluid intake or drinking pattern since the start of pregnancy?**
Yes. Now I drink everything. Coke, orange, I've cut down on tea, I drink anything sweet.

2e. **Do you know what fluid requirements are recommended when you are pregnant?**
No.

Maintenance of a Balance between Rest and Activity

3a. **Will you describe your usual pattern of daily activity (how you spend a normal day)?**
Up at 6 a.m. to "feed the kids breakfast" then back to bed. 9 a.m, dress second child, do the shopping" I don't do any house work now. Before I was pregnant I was fanatic for house work" (Tears in eyes) "I'm too depressed, I won't even wash up". Allowed to weep freely.

3b. **Do you pursue any sports or undertake any vigorous exercise?**
Keep fit twice a week. Slimming club (Weight watchers) once a week (before pregnancy)

3c. **Does your job require you to stand for long periods or to be on your feet for any length of time?**
No.

3d. **Have you made any changes in your activities since pregnancy began?**
I've stopped swimming & going to "keep fit".

Maintenance of Sufficient Intake of Air

4a. **Do you usually have any difficulty with breathing or experience any periods of breathlessness?**
No.

4b. **Do you know how breathing may be affected during pregnancy?**
No.

Provision of Care Associated with Elimination Processes and Excretion

5a. **Do you usually have your bowels opened every day?**
No. Every 2 days. When on the diet, it was once a week if I was lucky."

5b. **Are you aware of any tendency to constipation or diarrhoea when you are not pregnant?**
Yes.

5c. **How do you usually cope with this?**
Senokot, two tablets every 3 days.

5d. **Did you have any trouble with haemorrhoids before you became pregnant?**
No.

Fig. 2.3 (continued)

5e. Have you noticed any change with your bowels or haemorrhoids since pregnancy began?
Not constipated now. I always get haemorrhoids when I'm pregnant.

5f. Do you usually pass urine without difficulty?
Yes.

5g. Did you usually have to get up at night to go to the toilet before you became pregnant?
No.

5h. Has there been any alteration in this pattern since you have been pregnant?
No.

5i. Are you aware of any changes that may occur with your bladder or bowel function now that you are pregnant?
Yes.

The Promotion of Human Functioning and Development, and the Desire to Be Normal
6a. How did you feel when you first realised that you were pregnant?
"Shattered". "I was on the coil". It was only $6\frac{1}{2}$ months since my little girl was born.

6b. How do you feel about being pregnant now?
"Getting used to it". "I haven't told anyone". "I dont want people to know. I'm afraid people will see me here and feel it's too soon". "I feel guilty because of the operation."

6c. What have you read or what do you know about having a baby and becoming a mother?
"Everything – by experience!"

6d. What do you think about labour and actually giving birth to the baby?
"I'm afraid of a tear. The wound broke down first time – it was an emergency, 2nd time the caesarean was planned. That was no bother", I'm afraid of the pain if anything goes wrong."

6e. How well do you think you (and your husband) will manage a new baby?
My husband will be thrilled. The Doctors say I definitely can't have another one (Caesarean Section). We wanted more children, but not yet, later on. I suppose thats being selfish. The doctors are going to tie my tubes this time. I'll have 3 children under 3 when this one's born.

6f. What are your views about feeding the baby?
Bottle feeding – same as the others.

6g. Do you know how to care for your breasts during pregnancy?
Yes.

6h. Do you know about the Parentcraft Classes that are provided in this hospital?
Yes.

6i. Do you plan to attend these?
No. I came the first time, when I had time. They were helpful then.

7a. What changes to your present life-style do you think pregnancy and having a baby will make for you (and your husband)?
It's awful. I never get outside the door now. I'm tied down already.

7b. How do you feel about this?
Not very pleased.

Fig. 2.3 (continued)

7c.   What family or other support do you have?
I've got good neighbours and a sister in Ireland. There's another two sisters living nearby but I'm not as close to them.

7d.   Are there any aspects of your religious practice that might be affected when you are in hospital?
I don't want to be sterilised – Contraception's different. That's not final – and sometimes it doesn't work. But sterilisation, it is final. It is not right. I know it has to be for safety, but I don't want it. I don't want a termination even if this baby is Spina Bifida.

The Prevention of Hazard to Human Life, Functioning and Interaction
8a.   Do you know what footwear and clothing are recommended while you are pregnant?
Yes.

8b.   Do you know how to care for your teeth and gums during pregnancy?
Yes.

8c.   When did you last attend a dentist, or when is your next dental appointment?
Two weeks ago.

8d.   Do you know what things or situations you should avoid in pregnancy because they might be a hazard or a threat to you and/or your baby?
Yes. Drugs, alcohol and smoking.

8e.   Have you taken any steps to avoid such risks since pregnancy began?
No problems to avoid.

8f.   What things would make you contact your doctor or the hospital while you are pregnant?
"If I were to lose" (blood from the vagina) "That's the only thing."

8g.   Is there anything that usually makes you feel stressed or anxious?
No.

8h.   Is there anything about having a baby or being a parent might do to cause you to feel stressed, anxious or embarrassed for example?
I'm stressed now. Only the operation (sterilisation during caesarean section)

Maintenance of a Balance between Solitude and Social Interaction
9a.   Would you say that you are the sort of person who likes a lot of people around you or do you prefer your own company?
Yes.

9b.   Have you ever been in hospital before as a patient?
Yes.

9c.   Have you ever been apart from your husband/children/family before?
Yes. Whenever I have a baby.

9d.   How do you usually react to being apart from your husband/children/family?
I'm alright if they're left with somebody I know I can trust.

9e.   How do they usually react to being apart from you?
Not very well.

Fig. 2.3 (continued)

9f. How do you think you will cope with being in hospital to have the baby, especially during labour?
Not at all. It's bad enough now. I can't imagine what it will be like then.

9g. How do you think your husband will cope while you are in hospital?
He'll cope. (said with determination)

9h. What is your reaction to being cared for by hospital staff and midwives whom you may not have met before?
Doesn't bother me.

9i. Do you have any views about student doctors or midwives looking after you while you are at clinic or in hospital?
No, I don't bother.

10a. How many hours sleep do you usually have each night?
About seven.

10b. Has your sleep pattern changed at all since you have been pregnant?
No. I don't have to get up at all.

10c. Do you know what rest and exercise are recommended during pregnancy?
Yes

11. Is there anything you would like to ask me?
When will I know when the baby's expected? Will they tell me the date of the caesarean today? I have to tell my sister in Ireland so she can book her holidays.

12. Midwife's subjective impression of the mother:
Looked tense, but generally her appearance belied her true nature and social class. ? due to depression.

12a. General appearance
Neatly dressed, rather overweight, wearing sombre clothes.

12b. Estimate of apparent intelligence
High – certainly higher than average for her locality.

12c. Personality
A caring, emotional and sensitive lady. Has high moral/religious standards, currently depressed.

12d. Social or cultural background
Comes from Southern Ireland. Social Class III.

12e. Language or difficulty with speech
Marked Irish accent – speaks freely.

12f. Any hearing loss, or physical feature of note.
None apparent.

Thank you very much for your help and letting me to talk to you.

The care plan (Fig. 2.5)

This gives the analysis of the mother's problems or, in Orem's terminology, 'self-care deficits'.

Orem's model was chosen because it was felt that her philosophy did not render a normal pregnancy 'abnormal' or problematic. It is considered that Noeleen's pregnancy to date was within normal limits but, as the history shows, there were problems and these have been identified on the care plan distinct from the self-care deficits they were felt to be causing. It is felt that they not only highlight in a concise and readily identifiable manner the mother's difficulties, but also show how the midwife might attempt to deal with these. This approach demonstrates the use by a midwife of information which is totally lacking in the conventional ante-natal record. Not only is the plan of care discussed with the woman, but it is available for reference by obstetricians and other midwives. Thus, in the absence of continuity of care by one midwife, the agreed plan could be continued and maintained by others.

The use of a care plan based on a model provides data for midwives to use in planning care for women and a nursing process framework provides an approach that is superior to that obtained from the conventional booking history, which is merely recorded on the ante-natal front-sheet.

Conclusion

The advantages of using a structured framework

on which to structure an assessment are borne out by this care study based on Orem's Self-care Model. The framework has been tested previously under different circumstances and with other nursing specialities, and therefore the model itself was not under scrutiny, but only its effectiveness for use in midwifery.

The systematic exploration of each system, biological, psychological and social, emphasises the underlying concept of the whole person and ensures the collection of comprehensive data, some of which might otherwise have been overlooked. The model emphasises the health state rather than illness, which makes it particularly suitable for use in midwifery, and as Aggleton and Chalmers (1985) point out, it is a model which consequently values both individual responsibility and argues for prevention and health education as key aspects of nursing or midwifery intervention.

Under normal circumstances it is unlikely that all five categories of care identified by Orem would be required by the midwife during the initial nursing process assessment of women who are potentially healthy and who are frequently highly motivated individuals already committed to self-care. These people require only the supportive/educative function of the midwife

---

Fig. 2.4 Sample Assessment Form based on Orem's Self-Care Model, incorporating the obstetric requirements of a conventional ante-natal booking history

Name	Likes to be called	Marital Status
Address	Next of Kin	Age
Phone	Relationship	Date of Birth
Ethnic Origin	Phone	Religion
Booking Date	Height	Community Midwife
Gravida	Urine	Other Investigations
Parity	Blood Pressure	

Fig. 2.4 (continued)

Relevant Obstetric History

Maintenance of a Sufficient Intake of Food

Diet and eating habits prior to pregnancy

Any change in these due to pregnancy

Woman's understanding of food and calorific requirements during pregnancy

Any specific dietary requirements due to culture or custom, especially when in hospital

Maintenance of Sufficient Intake of Fluid

Daily fluid intake prior to pregnancy

Any alteration in fluid intake due to pregnancy

Amount of milk/milk products usually consumed per day

Amount of alcohol usually drunk each week

Woman's understanding of fluid and alcohol consumptIon during pregnancy

Maintenance of a Balance between Rest and Activity

Usual pattern of daily activity/nature of occupation if other than housewife

Any particular hazards or problems related to her job during pregnancy

Plans for maternity leave and working after the baby's birth

Usual recreational pursuits

Any alteration in these activities proposed or already affected during pregnancy

Usual sleeping pattern

Any alteration in sleep pattern since the onset of pregnancy

Woman's understanding of rest and exercise requirements, and sexual intercourse during pregnancy

Maintenance of a Sufficient Intake of Air

Any breathing problems, breathlesness or fainting when not pregnant

Fig. 2.4 (continued)

Any effect on the above, or evidence of reduced activity due to their effects since the onset of pregnancy

Provision of Care Associated with Elimination

Usual bowel habit

Any change in habit since the onset of pregnancy

Usual method of coping with constipation or diarrhoea

Presence of any haemorrhoids now or in previous pregnancies

Usual pattern of micturition when not pregnant

Any change in micturition since the onset of pregnancy

Woman's understanding of the effect of pregnancy on the bladder and bowel

Promotion of Human Functioning, Development and Desire to Be Normal

Family situation and home environment, social circumstances

Home assessment by community midwife

Husband/partner's occupation

Woman's attitude towards this pregnancy initially and at present time

Attitude of husband/partner, other family and any siblings to present pregnancy

Woman's knowledge about health care maintenance during pregnancy and puerperium

Any special requests for the management of labour

Parents' views on and knowledge about infant feeding

Breast assessment

Woman's attitude to parentcraft classes and awareness of various classes available

Degree of family and other support available after the baby is born

Resources available and ability of woman and husband/partner to cope as parents

Any particular religious practice relevant to childbirth

General physical assessment

Fig. 2.4 (continued)

Prevention of Hazard to Human Life, Functioning and Interaction

First day of last normal menstrual period

Expected date of confinement by dates, examination, ultrasonic scan

Results of abdominal and vaginal examinations

Parents' views of alpha-feto protein test

Woman's understanding of other screening tests undertaken in pregnancy

Woman's understanding of situations which might be harmful in pregnancy, especially drugs. Any medications or treatment currently being undertaken. Any known allergies

Relevant medical and surgical history

Relevant family history

Woman's understanding of symptoms of onset of labour and other circumstances which would make her contact a doctor

Any particular fears or anxieties relating to childbirth

Maintenance of a Balance between Solitude and Socialisation

Attitude to care in hospital and ability to relate to others

Husband/partner's response to being present during labour

Likely reaction to separation by woman, partner, any other children

Reaction to being cared for by student doctors, nurses or midwives (for Moslem women, reaction to being cared for by male doctors)

Proposed length of stay in hospital after the birth of the baby

Midwife's Summary and Overall Impression Gained during the Interview

General appearance and behaviour of woman

Ability to read, communicate and understand English

Any physical disability, hearing or sight defect or handicap during pregnancy and the puerperium. However, the model also emphasises care of dependants and involves all the family and significant others in the overall assessment. This factor makes the model particularly apposite for midwifery, when the client may be a woman and a fetus, a mother and her baby, or, because modern midwifery is a family affair, the husband/partner, other siblings and even grandparents.

Orem's model is not only highly suited for use in midwifery but also lends itself to a nursing process approach to care. Assessment involves firstly the woman's ability to maintain her own self-care and secondly the ability of the midwife to decide in what ways self-care may be deficient and so identify a self-care deficit. By observation and discussion, the midwife should be able to recognise the particular lack of knowledge, skills or motivation for self-care displayed by the woman, or the effect of social or cultural norms which may be imposing their own limitations on her ability to care effectively for herself in order to maintain optimum health. By so doing, the midwife has already determined the extent to which she needs to adopt an supportive/educative role in order to achieve recovery of balance between self-care demands and self-care abilities in the woman. This is the principle behind goal-setting using the Orem model. Planning care therefore seeks to determine ways in which these deficits can be met in order to restore the balance.

The major emphasis of this model is on the necessity for the midwife to discuss or negotiate the setting of goals and the development of a care plan with the woman and her family. This partnership of care lends itself particularly to those couples who present at booking clinic with their 'birth plan' and individual requests for personalised care and management, especially during labour.

Orem sees evaluation of goals in terms of when the patient or woman demonstrates an increased capacity to perform self-care activities. As this is unlikely to be diminished to any great extent in normal midwifery, evaluation has to be made in terms of the woman's continuing ability to maintain her own self-care in relation to the demands of pregnancy or the puerperium.

Orem's model proves relatively simple to use and adapts easily for use in midwifery. It combines a nursing process assessment and the ante-natal booking history into a unified interview and documentary record. Figure 2.4 illustrates how an assessment based on Orem's framework may be combined with the questions asked at a conventional booking interview. For the small amount of extra time taken, an immense wealth of data and hitherto undiscovered problems and needs were identified. In addition, the woman appreciated being treated as a person and having individual needs or anxieties considered.

While it is not possible to draw a general conclusion from the analysis of only one woman's history, the example presented in this chapter illustrates a trend found in other care plans in this study. This would almost certainly be reinforced if other care plans were to be written from the other interviews undertaken.

Therefore it is concluded that the use of a nursing process framework based on Orem's Self-care Model is highly suitable for use in midwifery practice and could result in improved quality of care and a higher degree of satisfaction for women and their babies.

Fig. 2.5 Care plan for Noeleen's ante-natal care

Pro-blem No.	Problem	Self-care deficit	Goal – self-care	Action to be taken by woman and midwife (Supportive Educative)	Date for evaluation
1	Guilt due to present unplanned pregnancy (Actual).	Social withdrawal and negative attitude to fetus.	She accepts present pregnancy, holds positive attitude to fetus. Restoration of normal social interaction.	1) Allow Noeleen to talk through her reactions to this pregnancy. 2) Use her strong RC faith to encourage a positive attitude to 'a child that is meant to be.' 3) Noeleen to discuss the situation with her priest. 4) Noeleen to endeavour to share her feelings with her husband. If necessary, he will come to ANC next visit for mutual discussion. 5) Noeleen to endeavour to be honest and open about her pregnancy with her neighbours.	Next clinic visit in 4 week's time.
2	Uncertainty about first day of last menstrual period and therefore of expected date of delivery (Actual).	Frustration and inability to plan ahead.	Establish EDD.	1) Obtain careful menstrual history. 2) Make abdominal examination to ascertain height of fundus. 3) Noeleen to record date of quickening. 4) Vaginal examination by obstetrician to establish size and shape of uterus. 5) Ultrasonic scan to estimate development of fetus. 6) Discuss findings with Noeleen. 7) Estimate probable EDD and stage of present gestation with obstetrician and inform Noeleen. 8) Monitor fetal growth and height of fundus at each subsequent visit, and discuss findings with Noeleen.	Visit after 20/52 Each subsequent visit

Fig. 2.5 (continued)

Problem No.	Problem	Self-care deficit	Goal – self-care	Action to be taken by woman and midwife (Supportive Educative)	Date for evaluation
3	Weight gain of $7\frac{1}{2}$ lbs in last two weeks (Actual).	Compulsive eating and craving for 'anything sweet'.	She is eating a balanced diet of not more than 2000 Calories and not gaining more than 500 gm weight per week.	1) Examine reasons with Noeleen for her marked change in eating pattern. 2) Discuss her normal strategies for overcoming excessive eating. 3) Devise a mutually agreed plan incorporating relevant strategies to assist her to control her eating. Give a written copy of the plan to her. Check on her progress at each visit. 4) Discuss recommended pattern of weight gain in pregnancy and set mutually agreed targets. Give her a weight chart for daily weight recording, to be brought to clinic next visit for her progress to be checked. 5) Liaise with dietician for advice re calorie content of foods and diet sheet, as Noeleen refused to visit dietician herself. Aim to change her attitude gradually by positive reinforcement of dietician's help.	Next visit to clinic in 4 weeks.
4	Depression due to being pregnant and weight gain (Actual).	Tiredness and stated failure to care for her children, herself and her home.	Restoration of confidence and ability to cope with caring for children and home, i.e. keeping home clean and tidy, not allowing dirty dishes to pile up. Positive attitude towards herself.	1) Maintain a positive attitude re her ability. 2) Encourage her to maintain social activity despite stopping 'Keep Fit'. Involve husband in this. 3) Encourage her with her progress re diet and restricted weight gain. 4) It is expected that present depression will lift as her other problems are resolved, therefore concentrate on these first. 5) If necessary, investigate possibility of play school for other children. Liaise with medical social worker. 6) Monitor her mental state. If no immediate resolution or situation deteriorates, seek medical opinion. 7) Noeleen to contact ANC or own GP if she feels situation worsening or she needs support.	Next visit in 4 weeks.

No.	Problem		Goal	Nursing actions	Timing
5	Obstetric decision that she should be sterilised during third Caesarean section. (Actual)	Conflict due to religious conviction that sterilisation is unethical.	Resolution of conflict. No longer feeling guilty re sterilisation and inability to have more children.	1) Allow her to express her feelings. 2) Noeleen to discuss her conflict with obstetricians and her priest. 3) Allow her to reach an informed decision, without pressure, in her own time, giving support as necessary.	Next clinic visit in 4 weeks.
6	Fear of scar weakness due to a pregnancy so soon after her last section, and of pain and possible complications following another Caesarean section (Actual).	Loss of normal poise and serenity and inability to enjoy her pregnancy.	Woman aware of symptoms of scar tenderness and sure of action to take if necessary. Confident about her ability to cope with another operation successfully.	1) Check her past obstetric history, for evidence of wound infection or failure or scar to heal by first intention. 2) Allow her to discuss her fear and identify its source. Correct any misconceptions she may have. 3) Discuss cause of pain and analgesia available. If fear persists, identify low pain threshold as a specific problem near term and alert post-natal ward staff. 4) Discuss sources of infection and its prevention. Encourage her to eat sensibly so as to be in optimum health at time of operation. Mention relationship of stress and lowered body resistance. 5) Educate her re symptoms of scar tenderness and action to take if this occurs. Assess implications to the point she is ready to cope with them (e.g. admission to hospital and her arrangements for care of other children 6) She is to discuss her 'problems' with obstetrician for information and reassurance.	After booking clinic. 36 weeks of pregnancy. 20 weeks of pregnancy. Next visit to clinic in 4 weeks.
7	Possibility of abnormal fetus due to a) presence of IUCD b) family history (sister-in-law has 2 children with spina bifida) (Actual).	Anxiety and loss of composure.	Mother reassured by information regarding condition of fetus, and possibly fetal abnormality.	1) Obstetrician to discuss the possible risk of abnormality due to presence of IUCD after he has examined the mother and located the device. 2) Inform mother re results of US scan. 3) Reassess her anxiety level after this and discuss implications. 4) She is unwilling to have alphafeto protein test due to religious convictions. 5) Reassure her about state of pregnancy at each visit and reinforce normality whenever possible.	Next visit in 4 weeks. Each visit to ante-natal clinic.

Fig. 2.5 (continued)

Pro-blem No.	Problem	Self-care deficit	Goal-self-care	Action to be taken by woman and midwife (Supportive Educative)	Date for evaluation
8	Anxiety re care of children while in hospital (Actual).	Stress—affecting all bodily systems.	Relief of anxiety by ensuring provision of care for other children during her stay in hospital.	1) Confirm her EDD by calculation and by US scan—inform mother of dates (see No. 2).	30 weeks of pregnancy.
				2) Set a probable date for elective LSCS with obstetrician.	
				3) With her explore possible people available to care for children while she is in hospital.	
				4) She is to ask husband and sister in Ireland to book 2 weeks holiday over the time of anticipated operation so they can look after her other children.	
				5) She is to prepare children for her stay in hospital by spending a night(s) away with her sister nearby.	36 weeks of pregnancy.
9	Potential haemorrhoids.	Potential lack of fibre in diet and constipation.	Prevent recurrence of haemorrhoids.	1) Discuss fibre content of her diet.	Next visit in 4 weeks.
				2) She is to avoid constipation and take pre-ventative action: a) dietary roughage increased b) 2 Senokot as necessary	
				3) She is to report presence of haemorrhoids if they recur.	

References

Aggleton P & Chalmers A 1985 Orem's self care model. *Nursing Times*, 81, 1: 36–39.

Department of Health & Social Security 1977 *Prevention and health, reducing the risk: safer pregnancy and childbirth.* H M S O, London

Dickoff J & James P 1968 A theory of theories: a position paper. *Nursing Research*, 17: 415–435

Donnison J 1979 The role of the midwife. *Midwife, Health Visitor and Community Nurse*, 15, 7: 265–270

Downey C 1980 Adaptation nursing applied to an obstetric patient. In: Riehl JP & C Roy (Eds) *Conceptual models for nursing practice.* Appleton-Century-Crofts, New York

Goodman R & Gorlin R 1983 *The malformed infant and child.* Oxford University Press, Oxford

Henderson V 1966 *The nature of nursing.* Collier Macmillan, London.

Hinchcliff SM 1979 *Teaching clinical nursing.* Churchill Livingstone, Edinburgh.

King I 1975 *Toward a theory of nursing.* John Wiley and Sons, New York.

McFarlane EA 1980 Nursing theory, the comparison of four theoretical proposals. *Journal of Advanced Nursing*, 5: 3–19

McKinlay JB 1972 The sick role—illness and pregnancy. *Social Science and Medicine*, 6: 561–572

Moser C & Kalton G 1971 *Survey methods in social investigation* (2nd edition) Heinemann, London

Myles M 1975 *Textbook for midwives* (8th edition) Churchill Livingstone, Edinburgh

Myles M 1981 *Textbook for midwives* (9th edition) Churchill Livingstone, Edinburgh.

Oakley A 1979 *Becoming a mother.* Martin Robinson, Oxford

Orem DE 1958 *Nursing: concepts and practice.* McGraw Hill, New York.

Orem DE 1980 *Nursing: concepts and practice.* (2nd edition) McGraw Hill, New York.

Plant M 1983 Drinking and pregnancy, a cause for concern? *Research and the Midwife Conference Proceedings*, Glasgow 1982

Reilly DE 1975 Why a conceptual framework? *Nursing Outlook*, 23: 566–569

Riehl JP 1980 The Riehl interaction model. In: JP Riehl & C Roy (Eds) *Conceptual models for nursing practice* (2nd edition) Appleton-Century-Crofts, New York

Riehl JP & Roy C 1980 *Conceptual models for nursing practice* (2nd edition) Appleton-Century-Crofts, New York

Robinson S, Golden J & Bradley S 1981 A preliminary report on the research project on the role and responsibilities of the midwife: Part 1. *Midwives Chronicle*, 94, 1116: 11–15

Roy C 1976 *Introduction to nursing: adaptation model.* Prentice Hall, Englewood Cliffs, New Jersey

Schlotdfelt RM 1975 The need for a conceptual framework. In: PJ Verhonick (Ed) *Nursing Research* 1. Little Brown and Co., Boston

Stevens B J 1979 *Nursing theory, analysis, application and evaluation.* Little, Brown and Co., Boston

Sundeen SJ, Stuart GW, Rankin EDes & Cohen SP 1976 *Nurse client interaction: implementing the nursing process.* C. V. Mosby, St Louis

Thomson A 1980 Planned or unplanned, are midwives ready for the 1980s? *Midwives Chronicle*, 93, 1106: 68–72

Venables J 1980 The Neuman health care systems model: an analysis. In: JP Riehl & C Roy (Eds) *Conceptual models for nursing practice* (2nd edition) Appleton-Century-Crofts, New York

Walker J 1976 Midwife or obstetric nurse? some perceptions of the midwife and obstetrician of the role of the midwife. *Journal of Advanced Nursing*, 1: 129–138

Woolf P 1979 Maternal alcohol ingestion and pregnancy. *Midwife, Health Visitor and Community Nurse*, 15, 8: 308–310

World Health Organisation 1947 Constitution of the World Health Organisation. *Chronicle of World Health Organisation*, Geneva, 1: 19–43

3

Care plan for a woman during pregnancy, labour and the puerperium, based on Henderson's Activities of Daily Living model

Rosemary Methven

This chapter presents the plan of care used for a mother whose progress was followed from booking clinic in hospital until discharge from community care at the end of the post-natal period. Individual and standard care-plans for pregnancy, labour, the puerperium and the infant were based on Henderson's fourteen Activities of Daily Living (1966). The care plan was written as part of a dissertation for a higher degree in nursing. This means that the circumstances were somewhat different from usual midwifery practice, where complete continuity of care is rarely possible. Although the situation was unusual, it permitted exploration of the feasibility of using a care plan based on a model of nursing, and this experience will be evaluated at the end of the chapter.

A short discussion on the nature of health and illness in relation to concepts of nursing and midwifery precedes the reasons for choosing Henderson's framework. The limitations of her framework and the modifications necessary to make it suitable for midwifery care are presented, together with the actual record of care given to one mother and her baby. This is followed by a critique of its effectiveness in practice.

The concept of midwifery

Little has been written about midwifery from a philosophical point of view. Traditionally, it has been seen as a practical art, an act of doing, a relationship (Myles 1981). Walker (1976) isolated three fundamental concepts which make the midwife unique: the fact that she is a practitioner in her own right, the quality of relationship she makes with the mother, and continuity of care. Present managerial practice, which has segregated the components of midwifery into ante-natal care in the clinic, intensive or high-dependency care in the labour ward, and post-natal care in the hospital and at home, has interfered with the ability of one midwife to provide continuity of care for a mother. This must also have affected the ability of the midwife to form long-term relationships with mothers. Medicalisation of childbearing and a team approach to care in hospital and the community have further eroded the midwife's ability to undertake normal midwifery as a practitioner in her own right. Indeed, the definition of what constitutes a normal pregnancy and labour is now in doubt and some would even say that labour can only be considered normal in retrospect. However, the ideal persists and the current trend towards normalising childbirth and reinstating the role of the midwife are evidence of this (House of Commons 1980).

A nursing process approach to care is seen as one way of overcoming the deficiencies of the present system and enabling the mother to have continuity of care via an individual care plan. A midwife, however, would generally consider this second best and would prefer to provide continuity of care in person whenever possible. Nevertheless, the problem-solving approach to care should do much to enhance the credibility of the midwife and provide her with increased fulfilment in her role (Methven 1981).

Elements of Henderson's nursing model

Models of care reflect the author's underlying concept of nursing as well as her view of the patient as a person. Henderson's fourteen Activities of Daily Living are based on her classic definition of nursing (1966):

> Nursing is primarily assisting the individual (sick or well) in the performance of those activities contributing to health, or its recovery (or to a peaceful death) that he would have performed unaided if he had the necessary strength, will or knowledge. It is likewise the unique contribution of nursing to help the individual to be independent of such assistance as soon as possible.

This definition is inadequate, however, when considering a pregnant woman. Pregnancy is a state of normal, if altered health, and not a condition of illness (Methven 1981), whereas Henderson's concept of a person requiring 'assistance with activities contributing to health or its recovery (or to a peaceful death)' generally relates to illness and not to health; to sickness and not to wellness. Henderson's definition would then only apply to midwifery if the mother or her baby had serious complications, which would immediately take the primary responsibility for care out of the province of the midwife.

However, Henderson's definition does allow that nursing is assisting the well person in those activities which contribute to health, and this could be applied to helping a person maintain her existing health and preventing its possible deterioration. In this way, a midwife has a definite role in helping a mother to stay well in spite of the demands of her fetus and the physiological changes which occur in the pregnant state. Henderson herself certainly did not exclude childbearing from her thinking, for in another context she sees the nurse (and presumably the midwife) as 'the knowledge and confidence of the young mother' (Henderson 1966). The young mother could be said to have returned to a normal state of health following childbirth, but might still need help to maintain that state, and to succeed with feeding and other aspects of childcare.

In order to provide a satisfactory definition of midwifery care and of the woman during pregnancy and motherhood, a conceptual framework must be able to go beyond the usual and accommodate altered, though still normal, states of health as well as the education, emotional support and preventative aspects of care which are needed to enable a mother to remain healthy until her baby is born. In addition, a model needs to accommodate not only the changing state of the woman in pregnancy, labour and the puerperium, but also the totally dependent but neverthless healthy newborn infant.

It is for this reason that the term 'nursing' process has been used in relation to midwifery care, for Henderson's model is a nursing model designed for nurses caring for sick people, and not primarily for midwives caring for those who are well. It has been adapted for use in midwifery but cannot be said to be a model for midwifery. Therefore the term 'midwifery process' is felt to be inappropriate.

Some contend that Henderson's Activities of Daily Living do not constitute a model for nursing, and she would agree with such an assessment. In her book, *The Nature of Nursing* (1966) she sees her ideas only as 'concepts', a view endorsed by the Nursing Development Conference Group (1973). Henderson, however, must be credited with insight into nursing which was well in advance of any contemporary thinking, and which has provided a framework that has been developed by others and proved to be a foundation for later models of care.

Henderson's and Roper's models compared

Roper, Logan and Tierney (1983) consider that their 'Model for Living' definitely meets the criteria for a model of nursing. It may be said to represent a British interpretation of most of Henderson's earlier ideas. They have adapted Henderson's fourteen Activities of Daily Living into twelve Activities of Living thus:

assessment of the person, and fundamental to the concept of nursing process (Bevis 1979). Crow (1977) writes:

> If we believe man is a unified whole consisting of body, soul and spirit, that he is part of his environment, a product of his past, a social being with norms and habits and customs and one capable of thinking and feeling; then we shall want to take these things into account when planning patient care and thus ask questions about them.

Henderson (1966)

1 Breathe normally
2 Eat and drink adequately
3 Eliminate by all avenues of elimination
4 Move and maintain a desirable posture; (walk, sit, lie and change from one to another)
5 Sleep and rest
6 Select suitable clothing, dress and undress
7 Maintain body temperature within normal range by adjusting clothing and modifying the environment
8 Keep the body clean and well groomed, and protect the integument (skin)
9 Avoid dangers in the environment and avoid injuring others
10 Communicates with others, expressing emotions, needs, fears, questions and ideas
11 Worship according to their faith
12 Work at something that provides a sense of accomplishment
13 Play or participate in various forms of recreation
14 Learn, discover or satisfy the curiosity that leads to 'normal' development or health

Roper et al. (1983)

1 Maintaining a safe environment
2 Communicating
3 Breathing
4 Eating and Drinking
5 Eliminating
6 Personal dressing
7 Controlling body temperature
8 Mobilising
9 Working and playing
10 Expressing sexuality
11 Sleeping
12 Dying

From this comparison it can be seen that Roper *et al.* have merely refined the earlier ideas of Henderson and that, apart from 'expressing sexuality', there is very little original thinking in this aspect of their model. Expressing sexuality would not have been an appropriate concept in the early 1960s, even in America.

It also appears that the later authors have further emphasised the physiological and behavioural aspects of health essential to a holistic

'Expressing Sexuality' has obvious application to midwifery practice using a nursing process framework of care. However, 'communicating', though it does not exclude 'expressing emotions, fears, questions, and ideas' as specified by Henderson, does weaken the holistic scope of the assessment. The spiritual dimension is entirely absent from Roper's model and the capacity to learn, discover or satisfy the curiosity that leads to 'normal' development or health would seem to be particularly applicable to midwifery where the psychological, educational and spiritual aspects of childbirth are fundamental (Gaskin 1980, World Health Organisation 1968, Prince & Adams 1978). This is especially true if the woman is to experience fulfilment in motherhood and reach the apex of Maslow's (1970) hierarchy of needs. Henderson's conceptual framework is therefore felt to be far more relevant and meaningful when applied to midwifery than Roper's.

However, according to the definition of a nursing model given by Riehl and Roy (1980) the Roper version may come nearer to the mark than that of Henderson, because the British authors also include preventing, comforting and seeking aspects of nursing. While the first two of these certainly have relevance to midwifery, the total scope of the midwife's role is so much greater than this that to describe midwifery care only within these limits would be unduly restrictive and incomplete.

A care plan based on the model

The nursing process framework for the individualised care plan was based on Henderson's original fourteen Activities of Daily Living. These provided the underlying theoretical foundation on which the assessment of the mother was made (Fig. 3.1). In designing a history-taking form it was necessary to avoid duplication of facts already recorded on the existing obstetric notes, while still providing an independent, comprehensive account of the mother and her midwifery care. For this reason details of previous confinements are not recorded in detail, and are alluded to in the care plan only where they have relevance to the present pregnancy. Henderson's concepts do not give guidelines regarding the way in which nursing care using her activities of living should be carried out, except that the nurse (or midwife) is to be the substitute for what the person lacks to make her whole, complete or independent in terms of 'strength, will or knowledge', i.e. 'the leg of the

amputee or the eyes of the newly blind' (Henderson 1966).

In writing the present care plan, the role of the midwife has been interpreted as the educator of the uninformed mother, encourager of the fearful or anxious mother, deliverer of the child during labour and demonstrator of infant care in the post-natal period until such time as the mother is able to maintain her own role independently. The midwifery care given is that which would normally be expected from a midwife but is expressed within a nursing process framework using Henderson's Activities of Daily Living (Fig. 3.2).

I have devised Standard Care Plans for problems that may arise during maternity care, and these are used in addition to a woman's Individual Care Plan if continuing assessment indicates a need. Some examples of these Standard Care Plans are given in Figure 3.3.

Evaluation of the care given

Pregnancy

I was able during the ante-natal period to have full responsibility for the care of Jennifer and to see her each time she visited the ante-natal clinic. She commented on the difference this one-to-one relationship made and how much she appreciated its value and that it was possible to discuss topics with her to a depth not previously experienced in midwifery practice. For example, deliberate and specific investigation into diet, fluid intake and bowel action at the booking clinic disclosed difficulties and problems which would not normally have come to light. Many mothers display some dietary difficulties which need specific advice and many, like Jennifer, eat too much carbohydrate and too little protein and fresh fruit and vegetables.

At the time of Jennifer's admission to the Gynaecological ward for the second time her frequent, often non-specific minor disorders had caused her to be 'written off' by the medical staff and labelled 'neurotic'. This was most unfortunate and, had this attitude persisted, it could

Fig. 3.1 Assessment based on Henderson's Fourteen Activities of Daily Living

Communication of Emotions, Needs and Ideas (verbal or non-verbal)

General
Jennifer appears shy and slightly anxious. Has a worried facial expression. Speaks clearly. English is her mother tongue.

Specific
She and her husband long for a companion for their only daughter, Anne Marie, aged four. They are anxious that this pregnancy should succeed because the last one resulted in a right salpingo-oophorectomy at nine weeks due to a tubal implantation in April 1980. Jennifer was treated for primary infertility before Anne Marie was born, and has also had a spontaneous miscarriage at eight weeks.

Attitude to Pregnancy
Jennifer and her husband are both 'absolutely delighted'. There has been no previous contraception so she feels confident regarding the first day of her last normal menstrual period and therefore about her expected date of confinement. She is unwilling to have the alpha-feto protein test in case she should not conceive again if her present pregnancy had to be terminated. They do not wish to know the sex of the child until delivery. Jennifer appreciates the need to attend ante-natal clinic regularly and to telephone if unable to keep an appointment.

Attitude to Labour
Wishes her husband to be present for delivery, especially as 'he missed the last one', and they don't anticipate having more than two children. She does not mind witnessing students being present, if necessary. Would like an epidural to be given at the onset of labour because the last one was performed when labour was too far advanced for it to be effective. Jennifer would prefer a spontaneous onset of labour but is not opposed to induction. She had a Keilland's forceps delivery last time and does not hold negative views about another one. No other strong preferences.

Attitude to Puerperium
Feels confident about being able to breast feed successfully despite artificially feeding Anne Marie. Would prefer a five-day stay in hospital.

Relationships
All family relationships are congenial. Has a good rapport with the community midwife, whom she remembers from last time.

Posture and Movement
Has a slight stoop but walks normally. Height 5'5". Shoe size 6, appropriate for height, which suggests an adequate pelvis. No backache but frequent pelvic pain, possibly due to adhesions following salpingectomy in April 1980. All movements appear within normal range.

Diet and Fluid Intake

General
Appears healthy, of average build. Weight 51.10 kg, appropriate for height.

Diet
Normally high in carbohydrates and low in roughage. Advised to reduce bread, pastry, potatoes and sweet foods and to include more fresh fruit, vegetables and eat wholemeal bread and natural bran.

Fluid Intake
Generally low in order to reduce urinary output. Drinks alcohol occasionally.

Effect of Pregnancy
Slight nausea initially. Has decreased fluid intake in order to reduce the effects of physiological frequency of micturition.

Elimination

Micturition
Passes small amounts of urine frequently even when not pregnant. Needs to get up to the toilet once or twice each night. A midstream specimen of urine revealed no bacteriuria. Intravenous pyelogram in 1971 had a normal result. Jennifer is unsure why it was felt to be necessary.

Fig. 3.1 (continued)

Bowels	Tends to be constipated. Attempts to alleviate this by diet. Has had several haemorrhoids since her last pregnancy, which are painful when she is constipated. History of gastro–enteritis in her teens.
Vagina	History of stale blood loss at nine and twelve weeks which necessitated hospital admission. No abnormal loss at present.
Skin	No evidence of increased perspiration or rash.

Appearance and Personal Care

General	Evidence of normal bodily care, hygiene and attention to personal appearance.
Upper Trunk	Face slightly flushed. No evidence of chloasma. Breath sweet. Teeth and gums in good condition. Attends dentist regularly. No oedema of fingers. Nails clean and not bitten.
Breasts	Marked evidence of enlargement at eight weeks. Nipples normal and well protracted. Pigmentation minimal, could become sore easily. Evidence of glandular activity and colostrum secretion. Preparation for breast-feeding to be made by normal hygiene and gentle friction to nipple area.
Abdomen	Salpingectomy scar just above pubic hair line, livid but well-healed. Normal distribution of pubic hair. Feint linea nigra. Evidence of previous striae gravidarum.
Pelvic Area	Leucorrhoea only. Episiotomy scar healed by first intention.
Lower Limbs	No evidence of varicosed veins. No oedema palpable on ankles. Feet clean and well cared for. No epidermophytosis.

Clothing	Casually dressed – suitable for season and stage of pregnancy. Wearing a good, well-supporting brassiere with broad straps. No need for support stockings. Shoes low heeled and suitable for pregnancy.
Maintenance of Temperature	Normal temperature maintained. No evidence of thyroid enlargement.
Breathing and Circulation	Breathes easily and regularly. Rate normal. No cough. Does not smoke. Blood pressure 110/70 mmHg.
Sleep and Rest	Usually sleeps eight hours each night, though disturbed by the need to micturate. Feels slightly more lethargic since the onset of pregnancy. Not having an afternoon rest at present. Advised to have two hours each afternoon with her feet higher than her pelvis.
Recreation	No particular hobby, but enjoys decorating. Both Jennifer and her husband are DIY enthusiasts and plan extensive home improvements and installation of central heating before the baby is born.
Work and Accomplishment	Occupation: housewife. Husband is an underwriter for an insurance company. They are financially secure, Social Group 2. Jennifer is eligible for Maternity Grant only.
Worship	Both are Anglicans, but not attending church at present.
Learning and Health Education	Jennifer attended local grammar school. She attended parent-craft classes with her first pregnancy, but is less convinced of their value now. Has read several books and current magazine articles about pregnancy and obstetric

Fig. 3.1 (continued)

care. Has seen a recent television film on labour. Appreciates the significance of a low-lying placenta which was demonstrated on ultrasonic scan during her earlier hospital admission for threatened miscarriage. Knows when to come into hospital in labour. Described the signs of the onset of labour correctly.

Environmental Dangers and Injury to Others

Mother	Age 32, 4th pregnancy with one living child. Eyes normal, sight unimpaired. Hearing within normal range.
	Dilatation and curretage in 1976 following incomplete miscarriage. Earlier treatment for primary infertility. Last baby born by Keilland's forceps, birth weight 2.725 kg Artificially fed, now aged four years and healthy. Sexual relations unaffected by present pregnancy. Has not used the contraceptive pill. Willing to have a hospital confinement in view of high risk pregnancy.
Investigations	Ayres smear obtained during recent admission for threatened miscarriage— showed healthy cervix. Immune to Rubella. Phenylalanine levels normal. No evidence of syphilis. Blood Group: O Rhesus Negative. Haemoglobin 12.5 G. Imferon infusion required in first pregnancy to correct anaemia. Pelvic examination not done due to earlier history of bleeding per vaginam.
Family History	Nothing of significance.
Drugs and Nicotine, etc.	Taking Ferrograd Folic tabs 1 each morning to prevent anaemia. No other medication. Does not smoke.
Home	Lives in a 3 bedroomed semi-detached house with gas fires. Central heating to be installed. Community Midwife's assessment satisfactory. Journey to clinic made by bus, 60p return. No excessive strain on pregnancy. Anne Marie at playschool during clinic visits. Husband to take one week's holiday when this baby is born. Anne Marie will be looked after by Jennifer's mother-in-law when necessary.

have been detrimental to her care and the outcome of her pregnancy. However, because a relationship had already been established with the midwife, Jennifer was willing to talk about her problems and eventually the root cause of her anxiety was discovered. It was possible with this system of care to discuss the unexpected cost and extra effort incurred by extending their new home and the frustration of having to manage without a kitchen for so long. This was really the turning point in her pregnancy health. The specific plan of action regarding diet and her decision not to install central heating until after the baby had been born can be directly attributed to the use of an individualised, patient-centred approach. Without this, her poor health and unhappiness might have continued until the end of pregnancy.

It could be argued that housing problems and patient problems not directly linked to the present pregnancy or health are outside the role of the midwife. However, if Crow's (1977) definitions of assessment and the concept of nursing process utilising a holistic approach to care (of the whole person) are accepted, then those factors which impinge upon a person's emotions, and which may affect their social circumstances must come within the ambit of the midwife's concern and care. Jennifer's case illustrates this well.

However, some of her problems were still not disclosed, and after the birth she revealed that she had been 'scared stiff' that the baby was not normal. The threatened miscarriage, repeated scans for placental localisation, and her own decision not to have the alpha-feto protein test had led to this conclusion. Her inability to disclose her fear during pregnancy confirms the findings of the Royal College of Midwives Survey in 1966. It may, however, have been the assurance that the placental site was now regarded as 'normal' which had helped her to 'feel' better, and not merely the midwifery care. At the same time, her own enthusiastic response to the effectiveness of the plan of action for relieving cramp (Individual Care Plan 15) and diet (ICP 14) cannot be denied.

It is accepted that in a busy clinic there might not have been the opportunity to give the individual parent-craft instruction that was poss-ible for Jennifer. Perkins (1979) found that groups most in need of education about preg-nancy, labour and parent-craft are least likely to receive or recognise an offer of this kind of help. This suggests that alternative approaches are needed but at present research does not seem to have established what type and method of parent-craft education are best suited and most effective for the varied needs of different parents. Perkins (1979) also concluded that classes are not effectively offered to all who might benefit from them, a finding which was corroborated while caring for Jennifer. It was usual practice for a hospital parent-craft sister to talk to each mother at the booking clinic which Jennifer attended, but no precise record of that conversation was ever made except 'advice given'. The nature of that advice was never made explicit. Consequently there was a tendency for other midwives to leave all parent-craft education to this parent-craft sister but, as no provision was made for further meetings with mothers unless they spontaneously booked for classes, the poten-tial of the arrangement was negated. This was particularly so because the nature of the 'advice given' seemed to be no more than the times when parent-craft classes were held, and no individual instruction was forthcoming. It was found that this arrangement duplicated care given on the basis of nursing process principles, and in prac-tice the role of the parent-craft sister, as it was practised in this hospital, caused fragmentation of care and hindered the use of an individualised, problem-solving approach.

Trim (1979) found that parent-craft education significantly reduced the levels of medication required by women during labour. In view of Jennifer's past history and personality, her rapid labour on this occasion would appear to support this. Parent-craft education had reduced fear of the unknown and consequently her anxiety levels were lower. As a result, her physiology was unimpeded by adverse neuro-hormonal factors and labour proceed smoothly and effectively. Jennifer had chosen not to attend organised parent-craft classes, but had benefitted from instruction on a person-to-person basis, a method which is supported by the individualised approach to care used with nursing process.

Apart from the initial interview at the booking clinic, use of a nursing process approach to care did not take more time than a traditional ap-proach. At each visit, the plan of care was rapidly reviewed and any new or unresolved problems readily identified. Conversation began at the point where it had been discontinued on the previous visit, which also saved time because a relationship had already been established be-tween mother and midwife, allowing goal-directed conversation to commence immediately. Jennifer appreciated that 'the midwife knew what she was talking about' and that she 'did not get asked the same questions each time'. These findings correspond with the Westminster Hospital Report (Hogg & Hague 1980). Familiarity with the assessment form speeded up history-taking and, as the relationship with the mother developed, additional information could be added.

Labour

The same freedom and responsibility granted to me in the ante-natal clinic was not possible in the delivery suite and post-natal wards, so that strict adherence to hospital practice had to be followed on the whole. The administration of an enema was routine despite the findings of Romney and Gordon (1981) that this is not necessary in most cases. However, Jennifer met the criteria which did require an enema to be given prior to established labour, because she had experienced constipation in the previous few days and her bowels had not been opened.

Research into shaving of pubic hair yields varied results. Johnson and Siddall (1922), Burchall (1964) and Kantor et al. (1965) showed that there was no difference in infection rates between shaved and unshaved perineums. Perineal healing has also been shown not to be affected by the ritual. Patient satisfaction is much higher if the pubic hair does not have to re-grow, although long pubic hair does tend to become contaminated with lochia. The argument in favour of shaving is that, if an emergency caesarean section is needed, then the mother is already prepared. In practice a compromise operated at the hospital in question; the pubic hair was untouched but would need attention in an emergency, while the labial and perineal areas were routinely shaved, although Romney (1980) considered perineal shaving an 'unjustified assault'.

The post-natal period

On several occasions the care given was not that which I would have chosen, for example, keeping Jennifer in hospital for a further day (ICP 27). However, this decision was made by a paediatrician. Possibly a further day's stay was warranted in view of Jennifer's moderately heavy red lochia and sub-involution on the fifth day. The doctor on this occasion did not respond to the midwife's request for Ergometrine (ICP 28) but it is possible that, whatever system of care had been used, these decisions would have had to stand. Nevertheless, when one person cares for a mother consistently she may give a more convincing report to the doctor than one presented by the person in charge of the ward, who may not have examined the mother personally.

Measurement of the fundus in the post-natal period is a good example of the problems which task allocation can cause. It was hospital practice not to use objective measurement, but to assess the degree of contraction and involution clinically. For this to be satisfactory the same person must make the assessment each day. As it happened, Jennifer did not sustain a post-partum

haemorrhage, and this could have been related to the fact that she was breast feeding. Oxytocin released during suckling should keep the uterus well-contracted. However, in view of her low post-natal haemoglobin level of 10.1 G (ICP 25) a haemorrhage could have had serious consequences. It is felt that this problem was compounded by the transfer home to a different set of midwifery staff and different midwifery notes. If the care plan had accompanied Jennifer into the community, the community midwife could have been alerted to the sub-involution and heavy lochia, and preventative action might then have been taken.

Preparation of the breasts for lactation and feeding has largely been based on tradition and the available research tends to give confusing results. After studying the literature it seemed best to adapt the measures advocated in the care plan to the particular mother. Waller (1946) found that poorly protracted nipples led to engorgement of milk in the post-natal period, but studies by Atkinson (1979) and Whitley (1978) found that rolling the nipple in pregnancy caused less pain in the puerperium for mothers in one survey, while mothers in another survey experienced more pain. Consequently rolling the nipple is advocated only for those mothers who do not demonstrate naturally well-protracted nipples.

There is similar confusion over the effects of pre-natal expression of colostrum. For mothers who have heard about this and wish to try, there does seem to be the additional benefit of early competence with putting the baby to the breast (Gunther 1970). Jennifer's experience would appear to support this, even though the certainty of improved milk flow is not yet proven.

The use of Rotersept spray for preventing sore nipples was current practice in the hospital. Earlier reports that Hexachlorophane was absorbed via the skin surface and later ingested by the baby from the milk have been denied (Rotersept 1985) but the manufacturer's literature on the subject does not indicate any reference to specific research to support their statement. The active agent in Rotersept spray is Chlorhexidine, a similar substance with a different chemical composition. It is claimed that Rotersept will act as a disinfectant against gram positive and negative organisms and so reduce the incidence of inflammation and cracked nipples (Huysmans-Evers *et al.* 1966). However evidence (McFarlane 1980) has shown that by using Rotersept in this way endorphins are destroyed, so that the baby can no longer discriminate the smell of his mother's own breast milk.

Jennifer's deficient pigmentation suggested that difficulties might arise due to soreness of the nipples which could require temporary cessation of feeding to allow time for the nipples to heal. In the event, feeding continued without interference or discomfort to the mother, and without problems for the baby.

Conclusion

It was most satisfying to be able to follow a mother through from pregnancy to the end of the post-natal period, both in hospital and in the home. Though this would not normally be possible for a hospital-based midwife, the one-to-one relationship definitely appeared to improve the care given, even though this care was sometimes given indirectly (Leeson & Gray 1978).

Jennifer's progress was not complicated by obstetric or even major midwifery problems but she did display particular needs, and it is felt that the use of a care plan based on Henderson's framework made the management of these problems more effective. In some circumstances the problems might not have been detected, let alone treated, without this approach to care.

Henderson's model is based on the activities of a person. As pregnant mothers are usually healthy, their activities of daily living are largely unaffected by child-bearing, although breathing and elimination are physiological rather than behavioural activities. Because pregnancy affects every system in the body, a model which includes more physiological activity would appear to be most suitable. Recording of blood pressure, which is so vital in pregnancy, did not easily fit into Henderson's framework but has been included under 'Circulation' and attached to 'Breathing' though it cannot be considered an activity as such.

The order of activities listed by Henderson was rearranged to give a more logical presentation of data. A good interviewer does not necessarily adhere rigidly to a framework but allows the conversation to develop naturally. She will record the information gathered under appropriate headings when convenient. For this reason, the order of headings was deemed relatively unimportant. The titles used by Henderson to identify her fourteen Activities of Daily Living have also been modified in order to 'Anglicise' their wording and in many cases to reduce the specificity of their intention so that they applied more readily to pregnancy.

Use of the model did impose certain limitations. The fourteen Activities of Daily Living were not designed specifically with the pregnant woman in mind, and adaptation was therefore necessary. In nursing there is only one patient, while in midwifery the client may be a woman and her fetus, or baby. Because modern midwifery practice is family-centered, assessment often includes the father and any other siblings as well. This is particularly necessary with regard to past obstetric history and medical history for the detection of familial and hereditary conditions. The Henderson model did not accommodate these features very readily.

Some of the Activities of Daily Living in their literal sense (such as 'Breathe normally', 'Move and maintain a desirable posture', 'Maintain a normal body temperature', 'Work at something that provides a sense of accomplishment' and 'Play or participate in various forms of recreation') have only a limited application to pregnancy and child-bearing. Conversely, 'Sleep and rest' and 'Keep the body clean, well-groomed and protect the integument' are highly relevant, though often not dealt with adequately in traditional forms of care and history-taking. These topics also provide a framework within which relevant health education can be given at the booking interview (Methven 1982). In the initial assessment, certain advice relating to normal care in pregnancy has been included. It could be argued that such advice should form part of the care plan but, as it related to topics which fell within the ambit of normal midwifery, these did not constitute problems as such, and therefore did not require an individualised care plan. However it was felt that the generalised advice on the standard care plans could be helpfully made explicit.

Literal application of the model did result in many relevant areas not being assessed at all. It was tempting to obtain the information thought to be required in order to provide a satisfactory standard of midwifery care, and then to work out ways in which this could be incorporated into Henderson's framework, and not the other way round. This serves to emphasise the inappropriateness of the model.

The solution adopted was to interpret the headings with imagination and in some cases to add sub-headings. In this way it is felt that a comprehensive and workable assessment format was achieved. For example 'dangers in the environment' was expanded to include the woman's home and general environment as well as the intra-uterine environment of the fetus and the hazards that it could sustain from the mother through drugs, smoking and excessive alcohol, X-rays, Rhesus anti-bodies, etc. 'Communication with others, and expression of emotions, needs, fears etc.' was expanded to include the psychological responses to pregnancy and the modern tendency for parents to participate in decisions concerning management of labour and various screening procedures. Similarly 'Work . . .' was expanded to include social circumstances.

For a healthy individual, 'temperature' appeared to be duplicated in 'maintain body temperature within the normal range' and 'select suitable clothing'. However, it is felt that this comment would apply whatever specialty was used with Henderson's framework. It was also difficult to decide whether to include colostrum under 'Eliminate using all avenues of elimination' or 'Keep the body clean, well-groomed and protect the integument'. Finally, in view of the earlier discussion on care of the breast in preg-

nancy, it was decided to include this under the latter heading, which was also used to include other aspects of breast assessment.

The framework as a whole was adequate in the circumstances in which it was used, that is as an adjunct to conventional obstetric notes which included details of the woman's menstrual history from which her expected date of confinement could be calculated. It is difficult to see where such information could be included if Henderson's framework was used in isolation, although it could be argued that the model stands in its own right and that a model specific to midwifery which would readily include the collection of such data is not necessary. Additional information could simply be gathered in the same way as the address, general practitioner and next of kin are identified.

In this context Roper's 'Activities of Living' would appear to be appropriate, for their heading 'Expressing sexuality' could be readily used to cover the attitude of the woman and her partner to the present pregnancy, their previous and future contraceptive practice and intentions, sexual relations during pregnancy, and the reaction of both parents to the baby, in addition to other specifically obstetric details such as the first day of the last normal menstrual period.

Anything new appears cumbersome and awkward at first. Because adaptation of the headings was necessary, it took longer to complete the assessment form and some duplication of data occurred. This difficulty should resolve itself with practice and greater familiarity with the assessment format. It is also likely that information might be difficult to locate by others using the notes. However this danger would be readily overcome by incorporating significant data into the care plan, where they would be easily identifiable as specific problems.

In conclusion, it must be recognised that in this study it is not clear whether the benefits experienced by both mother and midwife derive from the characteristics of the model used, or whether they merely result from a nursing process approach to care which in this instance was based on Henderson's fourteen Activities of Daily Living.

Henderson's 1966 model has been shown to be effective in providing a framework upon which midwifery care using a nursing process approach to care can be given. However, some adaptation was required, and Henderson essentially only provides a framework for assessment not for implementation. As such her 'model' may be said to be an improvement on the practice of performing midwifery assessment which is not based on any framework other than tradition. However a model specifically designed for midwifery, based on health and not on illness, resulting from research into what information midwives really need in order to provide effective care for the mother, and enabling the midwife to exercise her independent practitioner role within the health care team, has yet to be developed.

Fig. 3.1(a)

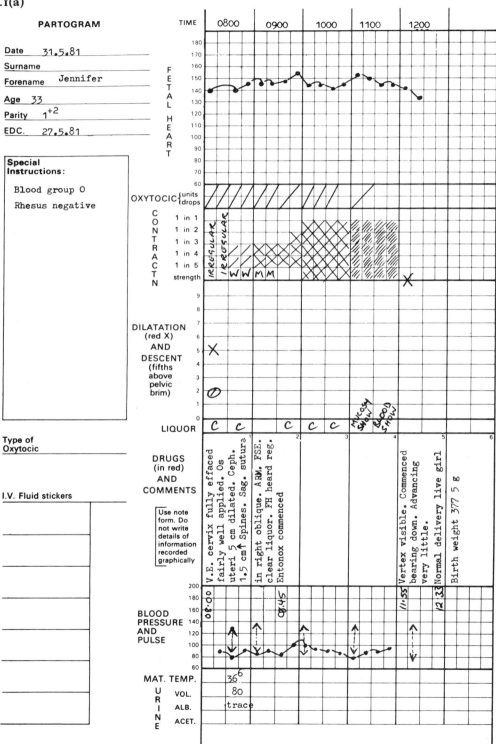

Fig. 3.1(b)

SUMMARY OF LABOUR

Mode
of
Delivery   Normal with episiotomy. Cord twice around neck and knotted

	Date	Time	Duration
Onset of contractions	31.5.81	0600 h	
Admitted to Labour Ward	31.5.81	0430	
End of first stage	31.5.81	1155	5 h 55 min
End of second stage	31.5.81	1233	38 min
End of third stage	31.5.81	1244	11 min
Membranes ruptured	31.5.81	0800	Total 6 h 44 min
Membrane rupture to delivery interval		4 h 33 min	

Admission to Labour Ward/Delivery   Interval   8 hrs.   14 min.

Type of labour   (Spontaneous) induced
                                       accelerated spontaneous

Indication for induction

Type of Membrane rupture   Artificial rupture of membranes

Type of Oxytocic

Type of monitoring   Fetal scalp electrode, cardiotocograph, midwife

Delivered by   student midwife   Indication   scarred perineum
Supervised by   Sister   for
                                         operative   episiotomy to prevent inevitable tear
Assisted by   Staff midwife   delivery
Paediatrician

Mode of delivery placenta   controlled cord traction; Matthews Duncan method of separation

Description of placenta appears complete   Complications   membranes torn and ragged
old infarcts present on amnion surface   of
Estimated total blood loss 200 ml   third stage

Details any post partum loss

Analgesia in labour   Entonox

Anaesthesia (if given)

Anaesthetist

Any other drugs given   Syntometrine 1 ml
                        Lignocaine 1% 5 ml

Any other complication
of labour or delivery

Post delivery condition   Pulse   80   BP 130/80   Temp.   36.14

ice pack to perineum   Epidural catheter   complete/incomplete

                          Cord blood   (taken) not taken

                          Swabs   (correct) incorrect

Fig. 3.2 Individual Care Plan for Jennifer during pregnancy, labour and the post-natal period

Date days/weeks	Problem No.	Mother's problem	Action to be taken	Desired outcome	Rationale	Evaluation date	Date discontinued	Signature
18.11.80 13 +/52	1	Safety Pregnant for the fourth time with only one living child.	Follow standard care plan for pregnancy. Doctor orders total hospital antenatal care.	Healthy mother and baby at term.	Mother 32 with only one successful pregnancy. Requires extra supervision and monitoring.	Each visit.	31.5.81	
18.11.80 13 +/52	2	Safety and Communicating Anxiety due to fear of losing this baby following stale brown loss PV at 9–12/52. Miscarried at 8/52 in second pregnancy.	Acknowledge risk. Explain action and rationale. Refer to doctor for opinion and ultrasonic scan. Report findings as soon as possible and establish cause of bleeding if possible. Mother to report any further bleeding immediately. Careful monitoring of fetal activity and growth and uterine size to detect possible placental insufficiency.	Mother free from anxiety and aware of possible reasons for blood loss and confident about stability of this pregnancy.	Decidua vera is sometimes shed at time of expected menstrual period. Placental separation occurring with threatened miscarriage can cause placental insufficiency and retard fetal growth.	Next visit 16.12.80. Scan shows low lying placenta (see problem 8). Fetus alive and active. Mother informed.	16.12.80	
18.11.80 13 +/52	3	Safety Risk of potential anaemia increased due to past history.	Follow standard care plan for pregnancy but stress correct diet. Remind about taking iron tabs. Observe Hb results carefully. Be alert for symptoms of	Avoid anaemia and maintain Hb level above 11.G through out pregnancy and puerperium.	History of fainting and anaemia in last pregnancy treated with Imferon infusion. Therefore increased potential for anaemia this pregnancy.	Monthly if Hb level above 11.G. 18.11.80 12.5G 16.12.80 11.8G 13. 1.81 11.8G 17. 2.81 11.1G 6. 3.81 11.0G 28. 4.81 11.0G	2.6.81	

Pregnancy and labour care: Henderson's model 57

tiredness or fainting.

5. 5.81   11.2G
2. 6.81 – Post
Natal Hb 10.1G
See Problem (25).

Date	No.	Need / Problem	Nursing action	Objective	Rationale	Evaluation	Date
18.11.80 13+/52	4	Safety. Rhesus Factor–Negative. Possible iso-immunisation.	Follow standard care plan.	Mother's blood free from Rhesus antibodies.	Once formed, Rhesus antibodies are a hazard for future pregnancies.	All results negative.	2.5.81
18.11.80 13+/52	5	Moving. Potential discomfort from adhesions from recent right salpingo-oophorectomy.	None at present. Be alert to possibility and reassure mother as to cause if pain develops. Observe for possible scar tenderness.	Pain free pregnancy – mother free from anxiety if pain occurs.	This mother hs likely to act on suggestion. Possibility of pelvic adhesions from recent operation. These will stretch causing pain as uterus enters the abdomen. Excision of tube is outside main uterine wall. Therefore rupture unlikely.	Each visit. 13.1.81. Pelvic pain causing discomfort. Plan activated.	7.4.81
18.11.80 13+/52	6	Communicating. Fear of possible multiple pregnancies.	Check routine ultrasonic scan for number of fetus present. Inform mother of result.	Establish whether single or multiple pregnancy at earliest opportunity.	Mother is herself a twin – other twins in family, therefore increased chance of multiple pregnancy.	Next visit. Ultrasonic scan revealed single fetus – mother reassured.	16.12.80
18.11.80 13+/52	7	Communicating. Anxiety due to inexperience with breast feeding (fed first baby artificially).	Follow standard care plan for breast feeding.	Mother successfully breast feeding a satisfied baby for at least 3 months.	Modern mothers are unfamiliar with breast feeding and require assistance.	First part of objective achieved by 12th post-natal day.	15.6.81

Fig. 3.2 (continued)

Date days/ weeks	Pro-blem No.	Mother's problem	Action to be taken	Desired outcome	Rationale	Evaluation date	Date discontinued	Sig-nature
16.12.80 16+/52	8	Safety Potential haemorrhage – placenta shown to be low lying on ultrasonic scan.	Explain possible cause of earlier bleeding to mother. Refer to doctor for further management. Explain implications of low lying placenta. Warn mother that further bleeding could occur. Advise her to contact hospital immediately should this occur. Continue to observe for signs of placental insufficiency.	Pregnancy continuing to term without further bleeding or danger to fetus.	Formation of isthmus at 8–12 weeks could have disturbed a low lying placenta causing bleeding. Further bleeding from placenta likely as lower uterine segment is formed. Bleeding painless and insignificant at first – can develop into haemorrhage fatal to fetus and mother.	For continual review. 16.12.80 Doctor ordered regular ultrasonic scans to monitor placental location. 24.3.81. Placental shift observed, site now normal in upper uterine segment. Mother informed.	24.3.81	
16.12.80 16+/52	9	Eating and Drinking Nausea – unable to eat or take iron – feels tired. Has not gained weight.	Investigate diet and cause of nausea. Test urine for ketones. Take blood for Hb check – see problem (3). Refer to doctor for possible change of iron tablets. Be alert for possible start of hyperemesis gravidarum.	Mother feeling fit and well – free from nausea and tiredness. Able to tolerate iron tablets.	Nausea is unusual after 14/52 pregnancy and could indicate early hyperemesis. Nausea is a frequent side effect of iron tablets. Tiredness could be due to hypoglycaemia or anaemia.	16.12.80. Urine free from ketones. Doctor prescribed Fefol (dose Tabs 1). Next visit 13.1.81. Hb 11.8G. Nausea resolved. Fefol tolerated well.	13.1.81	
10.2.81 25+/52	10	Safety and Communicating Unable to attend clinic as first child (Anne Marie) has mumps.	Assure mother there is no risk to fetus or pregnancy. Give Clinic app't. for 1/52.	Mother free from anxiety. Child well. Mother able to attend clinic.	Mumps not teratogenic and fetus now fully formed.	Next visit. 17.2.81. Anne Marie now back to school.	17.2.81.	

Date	No.	Patient problem/need	Nursing action	Expected outcome	Rationale	Evaluation	Date
17.2.81 26 +/52	11	Communicating Looks and feels generally anxious and unwell – multiple minor ailments.	Discuss pregnancy and social situation in order to find possible underlying cause. Continue with plan for problem (5). Advise 2 hours rest each afternoon.	Mother free from anxiety and happily pregnant.	Complaints genuine but trivial. Likely to be symptoms of a deeper problem.	Next visit. 3.3.81. Still unsettled. House in chaos due to extensive alterations. Sleeping downstairs with daughter. Continue with plan 7.4.81. Back in own bedroom. Looks and feels much better.	7.4.81
17.2.81. 26 +/52	12	Moving Cramp – mostly at night.	Investigate diet and estimate calcium intake. To include 1 extra pint of milk daily and ½lb cheese per week in diet. Mother to clench toes and dorsiflex foot when attack occurs.	Freedom from cramp and undisturbed sleep.	Cramp can be due to calcium deficiency. Contraction of opposing muscles is sometimes effective.	Next visit. 3.3.81. Attacks are less. Exercise gives rapid relief. Continue with plan.	
3.3.81. 28/52	13	Hygiene Slight oedema of both ankles.	Check activity level and rest periods. Check B/P level. Check Hb result. Examine legs for varicosed veins. Encourage 2 hours rest each afternoon with feet higher than pelvis.	Resolution of oedema.	Cause of oedema may be: back pressure from growing uterus, pre-eclampsia, varicosed veins, anaemia – see P3.	B/P 100/60. Not resting each afternoon. No varicosed veins. Next visit. 17.3.81. Hb. 11.G – warned to follow plan for P3. Oedema resolved. To continue with 2 hours rest each afternoon.	17.3.81

Fig. 3.2 (continued)

Date days/ weeks	Pro-blem No.	Mother's problem	Action to be taken	Desired outcome	Rationale	Evaluation date	Date discontinued	Sig-nature
17.3.81 30/52	14	Eating and Drinking Faulty diet leading to: constipation, bleeding, haemorrhoids, failure to gain weight, retarded fetal growth, falling Hb level, hospital admission req'd.	Mother will cut out sugar from beverages. Cook one main meal each day. Include protein, especially iron containing foods in each metal. Include more roughage as salads and bran flakes with cereal. Increase fluid intake by 1 pint per day.	A balanced diet giving a healthy mother and fetus free from minor disorders.	Kitchen being extended, no meals cooked. Eating only snacks. Acute constipation caused prolapse & rupture of Haemorrhoids. Mother thought bleeding from placenta and came to hospital. See Problem (8).	Next visit 24.3.81. Mother following plan. Enthusiastic about meals and effect on bowels. Continue with plan.		
17.3.81 30/51	15	Eliminating Haemorrhoids causing distress.	Examine haemorrhoids. Mother to replace after defaecation. Refer to doctor for prescription for Anusol Cream. Control constipation by diet as above.	Mother free from discomfort.	Anusol is an analgesic, antipuritic, antihydroscopic agent specific for the relief of haemorrhoids.	Next visit. 24.3.81. Haemorrhoids less painful, still need replacing after defaecation. Anusol giving relief. Continue with plan.	13.6.81.	
17.3.81 30/52	16	Hygiene Possible faulty hygiene predisposing to infection.	Discuss food preparation, cooking and storage methods. Investigate state of kitchen during alterations.	Safe environment for family and especially new baby.	Doctors suspected some gastroenteritis – past history – when mother admitted with constipation followed by diarrhoea. Correct any faulty technique now so new baby not at risk from salmonella.	Puerperium: Prior to and after transfer home. 3.6.81. Mother shown and supervised making a feed and sterilising equipment. 8.6.81. Assessed equipment and technique for baby care—satis.	8.6.81	

24.3.81 31/52	17	Eliminating Disturbed sleep due to frequency of micturition – mother has reduced fluids to combat this.	Obtain mid-stream specimen of urine. Palpate station of presenting part. Explain reason for frequency. Encourage fluid intake to minimum of 1 500 ml per day. Mother to rest for 2 hours each afternoon.	Undisturbed sleep.	Exclude possible infection. Frequency likely to be due to pressure from presenting part on bladder. A good fluid intake will prevent constipation and infection and promote good lactation.	Fetal head engaged in the pelvis. Next visit. 7.4.81. Midstream specimen of urine negative. Mother maintaining fluid intake at normal level but no increase. She is less anxious about disturbed nights and now resting for 2 hours each afternoon. Continue with plan.	1.6.81
7.4.81. 33/52	18	Learning Does not wish to attend parent-craft classes.	Discuss factors involved. Agreed to accept her decision not to attend. Give individual help each visit. Mother will read Parentcraft book, *Essential Exercises for the Child Bearing Year* by Elizabeth Noble (1976). John Murray Publishers.	Mother adequately prepared for labour and a new baby.	Mother is only just coping with upheaval due to house extension. Attended classes for first pregnancy. Rest will be of greater value.	Each ante-natal visit, during labour, and in the puerperium. 5.5.81. Mother appears to have good understanding of all topics covered. Has read book.	15.6.81
21.4.81 35/52	19	Communicating Anxiety due to failure of epidural to give pain relief in last labour.	Investigate reason for failed epidural. Discuss various methods of pain relief. Refer to doctor for possible elective epidural.	Mother free from anxiety and pain free in labour.	Fear and anxiety impede progress in labour. This anxious mother needs adequate pain relief. Epidural service available.	Epidural only given at end of 1st stage in first pregnancy. Doctor will review epidural when mother in early labour. Mother advised to come in early in labour.	31.5.81

Fig. 3.2 (continued)

Date days/ weeks	Pro- blem No.	Mother's problem	Action to be taken	Desired outcome	Rationale	Evaluation date	Date discon- tinued	Sig- nature
19.5.81 39/52	20	Eating and Drinking Inadequate weight gain since 21.4.81–500 g.	Investigate diet and activity level. Palpate abdomen to assess girth, fundal height, amount of liquor, size and activity of fetus. Refer to last ultrasonic scan for fetal growth. Refer to doctor for opinion.	Healthy placenta and satisfactory fetal growth until delivery.	Poor maternal weight gain at term may indicate placental insufficiency and retarded fetal growth. Induction of labour may be necessary if infant light for dates.	Mother eating mostly salads. Still overactive. Trying to complete alterations to house before delivery. Fetus active and feels a good size. Liquor amount normal. Fundus and girth consistent with gestation. Growth normal on scan. No action by doctor. For review next week. 26.5.81. Continue with plan.	31.5.81	
31.5.81 41 + /52 08.00 hrs labour	21	Eliminating Acute constipation for 48 hours prior to onset of labour.	Make abdominal examination. Make vaginal examination. Give disposable enema. Explain reason for feeling constipated in labour to Mother. Follow standard care plan for labour.	Rectum empty and mother free from discomfort.	An empty rectum allows greater freedom for descent of fetal head. Feeling of constipation may be due to pressure of fetal head on sacral nerves and rectum. An inhibited mother will not push well in second stage.	Enema effective. Mother still feels constipated despite explanation.	31.5.81	
31.5.81 41 + 52	22	Hygiene Delay in 2nd stage	Explain situation and action to mother.	Sufficient outlet to allow passage	Delay may cause fetal distress.	The next contraction.	13.6.81	

12.20 hrs labour		of labour due to scarred perineum failing to stretch.	Infiltrate perineum with 5 ml 1% Lignocaine. Perform right mediolateral episiotomy.	of fetal head without delay or unintended trauma.	Overstretching of perineum may cause uterine prolapse later on. A controlled cut heals better and is unlikely to extend.	Daily examination during first 10 days of post natal period.	
1.6.81 1st P/N day	23	Communicating Upset – due to daughter's distress at leaving her mother in hospital.	Visiting by Anne-Marie to be encouraged each day. Mother to make a fuss of her during visiting. Explain child's concept of separation at 3 years of age. Father to read special bedtime story.	Happy contented mother and daughter.	Mother's display of emotion likely to be increased due to hormonal activity and early 'third day blues'. A child of 3 years still vulnerable to separation but secure with father. See Bowlby (1963).	Next visiting time.. 2.6.81 Anne-Marie greeted mother warmly. Less upset on departure. Is behaving normally at home. Mother reassured.	3.6.81
2.6.81 2nd P/N day	24	Hygiene Nipples pink and slightly tender especially on right side.	Examine nipples before each feed. Supervise feed to ensure correct technique. Apply Rotersept spray as directed. Discontinue breastfeeding temporarily if tenderness increases or cracks become likely.	Intact nipples that do not cause pain during breast feeding.	Chlorhexidine Gluconate is a disinfectant and reduces the risk of inflammation and formation of cracked nipples.	Daily examination. 4.6.81. Nipples still pink but less tender. Continue with plan. 6.6.81. Nipples comfortable.	6.6.81

Continued

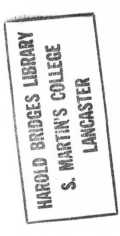

Fig. 3.2 (continued)

Date days/ weeks	Pro- blem No.	Mother's problem	Action to be taken	Desired outcome	Rationale	Evaluation date	Date discon- tinued	Sig- nature
2.6.81 2nd P/N day	25	<u>Safety</u> Post-natal Haemoglobin result only 10.1G.	Check delivery blood loss and present lochia. Refer to doctor for opinion and action. Encourage diet high in iron containing foods. Full blood count. Doctor prescribed Ferrograd Folic tabs and Ascorbic Acid 50 ml daily for 28 days. Confirm post-natal clinic appointment.	Haemoglobin level above 11.6G.	Untreated post-partum anaemia can lead to infection, diminished lactation, tiredness, irritability with family. Ascorbic acid assists absorption of iron in the intestine.	Blood loss at delivery 200 ml. Lochia quite heavy and red. Repeat Hb 9.9G by full blood count. Recheck Hb at post-natal clinic.		
2.6.81 2nd P/N day	26	<u>Safety</u> Baby appears jaundiced.	Refer to paediatrician. Discuss implications with mother. Institute modified demand feeding. Mother to offer 30 ml sterile water after each feed. Doctor requests 3 hourly breast feeds. Doctor will take blood for daily serum bilirubin estimation.	Maintain baby's serum bilirubin level below 12–15 mg per 100 ml.	Time of appearance suggests cause is physiological due to breakdown of excess fetal red blood cells. Glucuronyl Transferase is sometimes insufficient causing delay in bilirubin excretion apparent jaundice. Serum bilirubin levels above 15 mg per 100 ml (250 μ mol/l) kernicterus. A jaundiced baby is often sleepy. Extra fluids are needed to dilute serum bilirubin concentration.	Tomorrow. 3.6.81. SB result 174 μmol per 100 ml. 4.6.81. SB 169 μmol per 100 ml. Continue with plan for 1 more day. 5.6.81. Jaundice fading. Baby feeding well. Mother reassured.	5.6.81	

Date	No.	Problem	Nursing action	Goal	Rationale	Evaluation	Date
5.6.81 5th P/N day	27	**Safety** Baby passing loose, frequent, non-offensive stools. Possible infection.	Extra fluids discontinued unless baby hungry. Mother to reduce intake of fresh fruit and control constipation with other roughage, e.g. bran. Send stool specimen for culture. Observe baby for other signs of infection. Alert mother to risk of cross infection – not necessary to isolate baby yet. Doctor delayed mother's return home until stool result known.	Mother's diet suitable for breastfeeding while still regulating her bowel action.	Breast milk is influenced by mother's diet. Grapes and other fruit known to cause loose stools in infant. Possiblity of gastro-intestinal infection. Must be excluded. See Problem (16).	Tomorrow. 6.6.81. Stool report shows no growth of pathogenic organisms. Baby feeding and looking well. Stools still loose. Continue with plan.	8.6.81
5th P/N day	28	**Eliminating** Persistent, moderately heavy, red lochia.	Palpate uterus – assess contraction and involution. Refer to doctor and suggest course of prophylactic oral Ergometrine.	Lochia diminishing and uterus involuting normally.	Possible retained products delay involution and healing of placental site. Could lead to infection and 2° postpartum haemorrhage. Oral Ergometrine would assist contraction and expel any retained products aiding involution.	Uterus well contracted (mother breast feeding). Doctor declined to prescribe Ergometrine and said lochia was due to breast feeding and effect of Oxytocinon.	

Continued

Fig. 3.2 (continued)

Date days/ weeks	Pro- blem No.	Mother's problem	Action to be taken	Desired outcome	Rationale	Evaluation date	Date discon- tinued	Sig- nature
7.6.81 7th P/N day	29	Eliminating and Communicating. Anxiety after passing large clot containing membrane. Safety Potential 2° post-partum haemorrhage.	Mother called Community midwife. Examine abdomen to pal-pate fundus and rub up a contraction. Examine lochia and clot saved by mother. Reassure mother that fundus now well contrac-ted and lochia normal. Inform General Practitioner.	Uterus free from any re-tained products of conception and involuting normally. Mother free from anxiety	Retained placenta or membrane may cause secondary post-partum haemorrhage and will delay involution of the uterus.	G.P. – visited and prescribed course of Oral Ergometrine. Each visit. 8.6.81. Uterus well con-tracted, lochia, brown and decreasing 12.6.81. Uterus not pal-pable. Lochia creamy and mi-nimal. Ergometrine completed.	12.6.81 12.6.81.	
8.6.81. 8th P/N day			Mother to take Oral Ergometrine 500 g t.d.s. for 3 days.					
15.6.81. 15th P/N day	30	Safety and Communicating Concerned about rash on baby's forearm. Possible infection.	Mother called midwife. Make top to toe examin-ation of baby. Enquire re feeding and weight again. Examine affected area. Assure mother that baby's general condition is good. Advise mother to apply white spirit to pustules and keep arm away from baby's eyes and mouth. Discontinue white spirit. Apply baby oil to lub-ricate skin.	Mother free from anxiety. Baby free from infection.	Superficial localised infection not affecting baby's general health. Keep area dry to pre-vent spread. Avoid contamination of other vulnerable areas. White spirit is an evaporating lotion and was available in the home. Possibly due to abra-sion from identiband which mother did not remove until 12.6.81.	Slightly reddened area about 3 cm in diameter on baby's left forearm. One small pustule and evidence of several ruptured lesions. Tomorrow. 16.6.81. Remaining pus-tuled has ruptured, area slightly less pink. Continue with plan. Tomorrow. 17.6.81. No sign of infection – skin rather dry (due to effect of spirit) 20.6.81. Area well healed.	20.6.81	

Fig. 3.3 Some examples of Standard Care Plans for problems arising during maternity care

Date days/ weeks	Pro-blem No.	Mother's potential problem	Action to be taken	Desired outcome	Rationale	Evaluation date
Booking clinic	1	Possible Rhesus iso-immunisation	Take blood to establish if Rhesus factor present. If blood is Rhesus negative follow appropriate care plan.	Mother's blood free from atypical antibodies which may cross the placenta and affect the fetus.	Previous blood transfusion may produce atypical, cold antibodies. Fetal Rh. positive red cells entering maternal circulation cause harmful Rh. antibodies to develop.	Next visit
Booking clinic and subsequent visits	2	Potential hydraemia	Investigate: Normal diet and advise *re* food with high iron content. Mother to take routine iron preparation prescribed by doctor. Take blood for full blood count at Booking Clinic. Take blood for Hb. estimation each month – if result remains above 11G. If result is below this level, refer to doctor and devise individual care plan. Observe for signs of clinical anaemia at each visit.	Mother's haemoglobin level to remain well above 11G throughout pregnancy. Preferably without iron supplements.	Physiological anaemia in pregnancy occurs due to 25% increase in volume with only 13% increase in cells. A fall by 19 from normal Hb. level can be expected. Anaemia causes tiredness, irritability, increased infection, post-partum haemorrhage, thromboembolic disorders, poor lactation. Prophylactic iron and Folic Acid reduces incidence of anaemia in pregnancy.	Every month 3rd day of puerperium
Booking clinic and subsequent visits	3	Possible asymptomatic bacteriuria	Obtain MSSU for culture and sensitivity. If result over 100 000 organisms per ml refer to doctor for antibiotic prescription. Advise mother to drink a minimum of 1500 ml per day. Test urine for protein and note any odour at each subsequent visit. Observe for signs and symptoms of overt urinary tract infection.	Renal tract free from infection. Functioning normally during pregnancy and labour and after delivery.	11 per cent incidence of mothers have over 100 000 organisms per ml in their urine. Asymptomatic bacteria may cause acute pyelonephritis, anaemia, prematurity, light for dates infant, renal impairment. Incidence of pyelonephritis is reduced by treatment with short-term chemoterapy or sulphonamides.	Each visit

References

Atkinson LD 1979 Pre-natal nipple conditioning for breast feeding. *Nursing Research,* September/October: 267–271.

Bevis EO 1979 Nursing in the health care delivery system. In: F L Bower and E O Bevis (Eds) *Fundamentals of Nursing Practice.* Mosby, St. Louis.

Bowlby J 1963 *Childcare and the growth of love.* Penguin Books, Middlesex.

Burchall RC 1964 Pre-delivery removal of pubic hair. *Obstetrics and Gyneocology,* **24**: 234–237.

Crow J 1977 Nursing process 1. Theoretical background. *Nursing Times,* **16**, 6: 273–274.

Gaskin IM 1980 *Spiritual midwifery.* The Book Publishing Co., Summertown, USA.

Gunther M 1970 *Infant feeding.* Methuen and Co., London.

Henderson V 1966 *The nature of nursing.* Collier Macmillan, London.

Hogg C & Hague J 1980 *Maybe I didn't ask—the experiences of women having their babies at Westminster Hospital.* Community Health Council, London.

House of Commons 1980 *Second report of the social services committee, perinatal and neonatal mortality,* Vol 1 (Short Report) H M S O, London.

Huysmans-Evers *et al.* 1966 *Nederl. T. Geneesk,* **40**: 108. In: *Rotersept spray, an aid to breast feeding.* Roterpharma Limited, Middlesex.

Johnson R & Siddall RS 1922 Is the usual method of preparing patients for delivery beneficial or necessary? *American Journal of Obstetrics and Gynecology,* 4: 645–650.

Kantor HI, Rember R, Tabio P & Buchanor R 1965 The value of shaving the pudendal-perineal area in delivery preparation. *Obstetrics and Gynaecology,* **25**: 509–512.

Leeson J & Gray J 1978 *Women and medicine.* Tavistock, London.

Maslow AH 1970 *Motivation and personality* (2nd edition) Harper and Row, New York.

McFarlane A 1980 *The psychology of childbirth.* Fontana, London.

Methven RC 1981 *The process of childbirth.* Unpublished DANS Dissertation, Manchester.

Methven RC 1982 *An Investigation into the Content and Process of the Ante-natal Booking Interview.* Unpublished MSc Thesis, Manchester.

Myles M 1981 *Textbook for midwives* (9th Edition) Churchill Livingstone, Edinburgh.

Nursing Development Conference Group 1973 *Concept formalisation in nursing.* Little Brown and Co., Boston.

Perkins EM 1979 And did you go to classes, Mrs Brown? Leverhulme Health Education Project, Nottingham, 1978. In: *Midwives Chronicle,* **91**, 1091: 422–425.

Prince J & Adams ME 1978 *Minds, mothers and midwives.* Churchill Livingstone, Edinburgh.

Riehl JP & Roy C 1980 *Conceptual models for nursing practice.* Appleton-Century-Crofts, New York.

Romney M & Gordon H 1981 Is your enema really necessary? *British Medical Journal,* 28, 2: 1269–1271.

Romney ML 1980 Pre delivery shaving: an unjustified assault? *Journal of Obstetrics and Gynaecology,* 1: 33–35.

Rotersept 1985 *Rotersept spray, an aid to breast feeding.* Roterpharma, Middlesex.

Roper N, Logan W & Tierney A 1983 *Essentials of nursing.* Churchill Livingstone, Edinburgh.

Royal College of Midwives 1966 *Preparation for parenthood.* Royal College of Midwives, London.

Trim MM 1979 Pre-natal education evaluation. *Nursing Research,* **28**, 6: 38–42.

Walker J 1976 Midwife or obstetric nurse? some perceptions of the midwife and obstetrician on the role of the midwife. *Journal of Advanced Nursing,* 1: 29–38.

Waller H 1946 The early failure of breast feeding, clinical study of its causes and their prevention *Archives of Diseases of Children,* **21**, 3: 1–12.

Whiteley N 1978 Preparation for breast feeding – one year follow-up of thirty-four nursing mothers. *Journal of Gynaecological Nursing*, May-June, 7: 44–48.

World Health Organisation 1968 Constitution of the World Health Organisation. *Chronicle of the World Health Organisation*, 1: 29–34.

4

Care plan for a woman in labour and her baby, based on Roper's Activities of Living model

Marian McDonald

The care plan in this chapter is based on the 'model' for nursing developed by Roper, Logan and Tierney (1980) and describes the care given to a 22 year old woman admitted to the consultant obstetric unit of a busy maternity hospital. The client whose care is described is Jeanette Turner, who is pregnant for the second time. Jeanette has been married for $3\frac{1}{2}$ years and is in good health apart from her 'smoker's cough' – she smokes between 10 and 15 cigarettes a day. She is understandably anxious about her pregnancy because she gave birth to a microcephalic baby just over 2 years ago. The baby, who also had congenital cataracts, died at 3 months of age. Jeanette's present pregnancy, however, progresses normally and she has an uncomplicated delivery. She and her husband, who stays with her during her labour, are immensely happy and relieved to have a healthy baby girl.

Florence Nightingale said in 1859 that 'the hospital shall do the patient no harm' (Nightingale 1974). The majority of women have never had cause to be admitted to hospital until they are in labour but, as a result of alterations in maternity health services in the last decade, they are encouraged to enter hospital for childbirth. Hospitals are disease- and cure-oriented centres and the maternity client thus involuntarily assumes the sick role even though she is passing through a normal physiological process (Parsons 1952). Midwifery practitioners must emphasise in their care planning the fact that pregnancy and labour are natural activities of living, even when

they take place in the unnatural, clinical setting of a hospital. Above all, they must ensure that the hospital does the client no harm.

The midwife, 'a practitioner in her own right. . . .' (Central Midwives' Board 1983a), has a code of practice which prescribes her specific role in caring for the client. She must ensure that supervision, care and advice are given to women in labour, ensure continuity of care, and accept responsibility for the care being given. The role of the midwife includes preventive care, the detection of abnormal conditions in the mother and baby, and health counselling and education for the client, family and community at large (Central Midwives' Board 1983b). Roper, Logan and Tierney's model encompasses all the requirements of maintaining childbearing as a natural phenomenon and yet accentuates the midwife's prescribed role in caring for the client.

Elements of Roper's nursing model

The nursing care plan in this chapter shows that midwives can function well using this model, as it emphasises prevention of ill health and promotion of health, as well as the traditional concern with care of the sick. The twelve Activities of Living, shown on the assessment sheet (Fig. 4.1) are aimed at preventing potential problems from becoming actual ones. This allows the midwife enormous scope for health teaching as part of nursing intervention. The model also includes several dimensions which affect the Activities of Living, such as the client's stage of development on a lifespan continuum from birth to death, and the degree of independence or dependence she has reached. These dimensions provide a sufficiently detailed framework for all clients receiving care, be they newborn infants or maternity clients requiring antenatal, intrapartum or postnatal nursing care.

The Activities of Living (AL) 'model' incorporates the process of nursing framework, which is defined as 'the key to individualised care, heralding power to the patient' (Roper, Logan & Tierney 1980). This quotation has particular relevance for maternity care today, when clients are more active in asserting their rights to determine the type of care they wish to have. The submission of a petition to Parliament in 1983 calling for parents' rights to be defined in law and the publication of a booklet entitled *Denial of Parents' Rights in Maternity Care* (AIMS 1983) illustrate this demand for clients' rights to be respected. The nursing process is a method of organising the planning, execution and evaluation of nursing care (Webb 1980) and demands an individualised approach to care, involving interactions between midwife and client as well as a logical method of carrying out nursing practice, 'linking theory and practice' (Roper, Logan & Tierney 1983).

Carter (1980) states that the nursing process is based on humanistic principles and the current philosophy promoted within midwifery practice is that of family-oriented care which also reflects this humanistic approach. The humanistic perspective sees a person as 'a holistic, active, unique and meaning-giving being' (Carter 1980), this concept of holism being derived from gestalt psychology and from the work of Maslow (1970) and Carl Rogers (1951).

The rationale for the AL 'model' is based on a model for living which encourages minimal disruption of a person's usual living habits, fostering independence and self-help. The Activities of Living may appear simple, yet they have complex meaning which incorporate psycho-logical, social, cultural, economic and religious dimensions, the aim being to prevent the fragmentation of client care into separate dimensions. Roper, Logan and Tierney (1983) believe that people's values, attitudes, beliefs and temperaments influence their individual modes of carrying out each Activity of Living.

It is against this background and framework that the care plan in this chapter is written, with some adaptations to suit midwifery care.

Client assessment form

Roper's original form was adapted to suit midwifery practice. It was completed on Jeanette's admission to the labour ward, but it would prove equally viable for use on other wards within the maternity unit. A section for assessment of home circumstances was necessary, as many women request early transfer home following confinement. Feedback from the domiciliary midwife on the client's home and social circumstances widens the overall picture of the client and is used to complete this section. Accurate coordination of transfer dates and times is important and, as the form is intended to be utilised universally throughout the maternity unit, I decided to record this information on the assessment form (Fig. 4.1).

Assessment of Activities of Living

I used the format designed by Roper, Logan and Tierney (1983). This form was also completed on Jeanette's admission, and any actual or potential problems were identified from the information obtained (Fig. 4.2).

Standard care plans

Two standard care plans were designed, one for the client's nursing care throughout labour (Fig. 4.3) and the other for the care of the fetus/baby (Fig. 4.8), and both plans were formulated on the nursing process framework. All problems depicted were potential, and goals were stated, together with the appropriate nursing interventions. If the potential problems became actual, they would be transferred from the standard care plan to an individualised care plan.

Individualised care plan

An individualised care plan, which is shown in Figure 4.4, was designed around the framework of the nursing process, which demands from the midwife the ability to identify actual and potential problems the client may be experiencing on admission. Any potential or actual problems were taken from the assessment sheet and included on the individual care plan under the appropriate AL heading. Goals were then constructed, nursing interventions designed, and evaluation times decided.

Evaluation of progress

A blank sheet was provided to record the effectiveness of nursing actions and the client's progress (Fig. 4.5). A partogram was used to permit visual evaluation of progress and to record client and fetal observations, and this is shown in Figure 4.6. Any deviations from the norm would be transferred to the individualised care plan, acted upon and evaluated on the evaluation sheet (Fig. 4.5). A blank sheet was also used for evaluation of the baby's progress.

To assist interpretation of the evaluation sheet, a numerical and alphabetical legend is used for identification of the problems. The AL headings are numbered from 1 to 12 and retain their number throughout the documentation. Actual and potential problems are labelled alphabetically under their appropriate AL headings. Similarly, the potential problems on the standard care plan are identified by Roman numbers, for example:

2 Communicating   (a) backache less troublesome (individualised care plan)
                   (i) brief explanation of labour given (standard care plan)

Summary sheets

I designed two summary sheets so that a clear and concise record of the delivery and the baby following birth could be made, and these are shown in Figures 4.7 and 4.9.

Following the start of the second stage of labour, time is of the essence and planning nursing interventions under the Activities of Living headings as well as evaluating the nursing actions proved impracticable. A summary sheet allows more time to be spent with the client, and cuts down considerably on writing.

At times during the care, choices were made between alternative strategies. Where one course of action was preferred to another, a literature reference is given in the care plan to justify the decision.

Conclusion: review and critical analysis

In conclusion, I shall review and critically analyse the overall impact that the Roper, Logan and Tierney conceptual framework had when applied to a midwifery client.

Certain factors affected the way in which I interpreted and applied the conceptual framework, time constraints coupled with the necessity to reduce paperwork being prime concerns. These also influenced my decision to make adaptations to the documentation which I felt would enhance its impact and increase its acceptability in the midwifery field.

The labour ward is an acute nursing area, where the stage of labour in which a client is admitted and the duration and outcome of labour cannot be predicted. These factors inevitably affect the compilation of the care plan. In Jeanette's case, I was presented with a slow build-up of nursing care leading to increased activity as the birth became imminent, and I had no difficulty in gaining the desired information from the client. However in different circumstances, for example those of well-established labour, the procedure used with Jeanette would not be feasible. Consequently it would be beneficial to compile as much as possible of the intended care plan during the client's ante-natal visits, when time pressures are not so great. The care plan can then be reviewed when the client is admitted to hospital, and information updated if necessary. Not only would this save considerable time and cut down on writing in this crucial period, but any actual or potential problems relating to the client's Activities of Living could be acted upon earlier. In Jeanette's case, with support and health education, her smoking problem might have been resolved before her admission to hospital.

In an attempt to further minimise documentation, I devised two standard care plans, one related to care in labour and the other concerned with care of the fetus/baby. Standardising care plans does go against the philosophy of individualised care planning and could, if misconstrued, appear like routinised or task-oriented care. It is obviously not possible to cover every potential event in a standard care plan and there is a danger if the midwife uses it slavishly and does not apply original thinking and action in planning care. With these factors in mind, I formulated the plans upon scientific principles and research findings, and designed them using the nursing process format. The standard care plan, therefore, incorporates the four phases of assessment, planning, implementation and evaluation, and thus encourages the midwife to give individualised care and prevents her from using the plan simply as a checklist of routine care procedures. Roper, Logan and Tierney (1983) have the same views on standardised care planning. They acknowledge the usefulness of this type of plan and yet feel that standardised plans 'will need to be reliable, which can only be achieved by adequate trial, feedback and modification if necessary'. Finally, the standard care plan could prove a useful teaching aid for student midwives, as it links midwifery theory with practice.

As a result of the inter-relatedness of the Activities of Living, two items proved difficult to place under an AL heading. Pain, which is felt to be a normal aspect of labour, was placed under the 'Communicating' AL. In most instances the client indicates verbally or non-verbally whether she is in pain and often describes the type and degree of pain being experienced, and therefore 'Communicating' seemed the appropriate AL heading to use. Categorising the fetal condition presented another challenge. My reasoning that the fetus, whilst in the uterus, is in a potentially safe environment led to my decision to place fetal condition under the AL heading 'Maintaining a Safe Environment'.

Evaluation was the area within the care plan which proved most problematic. The unpredictability of labour makes judgements concerning times and dates for evaluating nursing intervention highly variable from one client to another. If the care plan is to be used as a teaching aid this may cause difficulties, as only by experience can a midwife decide when evaluation is necessary.

Maternal and fetal observations during labour require frequent monitoring, and I felt in this instance that a visual evaluation in the form of a partogram was appropriate, because it gave a continuous, easily-interpreted picture of labour whilst at the same time reducing paperwork. From the start of the second stage of labour, time was too limited to write the nursing interventions under the Activities of Living headings. To overcome this difficulty, I designed a summary sheet, which I feel is easy to understand and encapsulates the salient points of this critical stage of labour.

Finally, the care plan may be used as a legal document, providing a full record of all nursing interventions, and it also proves to be a useful guide to student midwives in developing communication skills.

When first encountered by midwives and students, the care plan format and documentation may appear threatening. However, with in-depth knowledge of the Activities of Living 'model' and with guidance and support, I believe that the advantages of the care plan far outweigh the disadvantages.

In summary, individualised care was achieved, and a one-to-one relationship did develop between myself and the client. The whole concept behind the plan, that of promoting independence and self-care with the primary aim of treating pregnancy and labour as natural activities and dispelling the perception of ill health, was realised.

In designing a standard care plan specially for labour, I felt I was covering new ground in that as far as I am aware no such care planning documentation has been published. I discovered that maternity care generates its own individual problems in addition to those described in Roper, Logan and Tierney's writings, not the least of which was my dual concern throughout all stages of the care plan for both the client and her fetus/baby. Only by constantly reviewing and refining the care plan will it prove to be viable and worthwhile both in theory and practice.

Fig. 4.1. Client assessment form

SURNAME: TURNER

OTHER NAMES: Jeanette Ann

LIKES TO BE CALLED: Jeanette

ADDRESS: 7a Ash Terrace
Billingham, Cleveland

TELEPHONE NUMBER: None

DATE OF BIRTH: 13.6.1961   AGE: 22 years

RELIGIOUS/CULTURAL BELIEFS: Church of England
(non practising)

OCCUPATION: Housewife

WORK PLANS: None

MARITAL STATUS: Married 12.8.80

NEXT OF KIN: Philip TURNER   RELATIONSHIP: Husband

ADDRESS: As above

TELEPHONE NUMBER: —

PARTNER'S OCCUPATION: Cleveland Transit Bus Driver

HOME CIRCUMSTANCES: Lives with husband in one
bedroomed
ground floor flat.
Centrally heated.
Awaiting rehousing
to council house
following baby's birth.
Mr Turner is a shift
worker, may have
problems visiting
—arrangements
made
to suit him.

ADMISSION/TRANSFER DETAILS

DATE	TIME	WARD
5.3.84	9.00 pm	Labour 4
6.3.84	6.50 am	Post Natal 3

REASONS FOR ADMISSION: Labour

GRAVIDA: 2   PARITY: 1 (died)   EDD: 1.3.84

RELEVANT PAST OBSTETRIC HISTORY: 1981 Full term, normal delivery of microcephalic infant with cataracts. Baby died at 3 months of age.

RELEVANT MEDICAL/SURGICAL HISTORY: —

DRUG THERAPY: —

BLOOD GROUP: O   RHESUS FACTOR: Positive

ANTIBODIES DETECTED: —

DATA COLLECTED BY:

Fig. 4.2. Assessment of Activities of Living

	Assessment of activities of living	Client's problems (a) Actual (p) Potential
1 Maintaining a safe environment	Usually independent. Familiar with labour ward surroundings. Requests early transfer from hospital – home surroundings assessed and suitable.	
2 Communicating	Rather quiet, gaining confidence in husband's presence (Ball 1981). Looks anxious, worried about this pregnancy in case baby is abnormal. Claims she can cope well with labour, does not wish an epidural (Moir 1978). Wants husband to be present during labour and delivery.	(a) anxiety over fetal wellbeing.
3 Breathing	Smokes 10–15 cigarettes daily. Has a cough she relates to smoking, non-productive. Not breathless on exertion. Tried to give up smoking but did not succeed.	(p) chest infection. (p) inability to use Entonox. (p) fetal distress due to anoxia because of nicotine effects (Spastics Society 1982).
4 Eating and drinking	Healthy appetite. No specific dietary likes or dislikes. Suffers from heartburn, which is relieved by sucking 'Rennies'. Social drinker 1–2 lagers weekly (Lewis 1983). No oedema Wishes to breast-feed baby. WEIGHT 89 kg HEIGHT 164 cm	(a) heartburn.
5 Eliminating	Regular bowel action daily. Bowels open that evening. Refuses preparatory enema in labour (Romney & Gordon 1981). Micturition normal, although goes more frequently because of fetal pressure on the bladder.	

Fig. 4.2 (continued)

Assessment of activities of living		Client's problems (a) Actual (p) Potential
6 Personal cleansing and dressing	Daily bath. Meticulously clean. Wears upper set of dentures (never takes them out).	
7 Controlling body temperature	Body temperature within range of normal on admission.	
8 Mobilising	Typical maternity gait. Requests to be ambulant during labour. No preference over delivery position.	
9 Working and playing	Has not worked since prior to her last pregnancy. Not planning to return to work. Likes to watch television.	
10 Expressing sexuality	Feels ungainly and will be glad to return to the non-pregnant state. No vaginal discharge.	
11 Sleeping	Sleeps well 8–10 hours nightly. Has an afternoon nap most days. Has never taken or needed sedatives.	
12 Dying	Previous baby died at 3 months due to microcephaly.	

Fig. 4.3 Standard care plan for a woman in labour

Potential Problem	Goal	Nursing intervention	Evaluate	Resolved
1 Environment				
(i) Wrong client receiving treatment due to mistaken identity	Correct identification and documentation. Criteria No mistakes are made.	Complete identiband with client's name and case number	On admission	
		Check correct case record		5.3.84 9 pm
(ii) Fetal distress due to hypoxia	Early detection of distress. Criteria Stable fetal heart rate.	Monitor fetal heart rate during first stage of labour	½ hourly	
		Monitor fetal heart rate during second stage of labour. High risk fetus; apply external transducers and acquire continuous ultrasound recordings of fetal heart rate (Schifrin 1979). Apply fetal scalp electrode following rupture of membranes.	Between contractions	
		Palpate fundal height, lie of fetus, presentation and descent of presenting part.	Hourly	
(iii) Spontaneous rupture of membranes due to increasing uterine pressure or no apparent reason	Ensure fetal well-being. Criteria No prolapsed cord, no meconium staining, stable fetal heart rate.	Observe for meconium staining of liquor		6.3.84 6.30 am
		Observe fetal heart rate	Immediately	6.3.84 1.20 am
		Using correct aseptic technique perform vaginal examination.	Following intervention throughout labour	6.3.84 1.30 am
		Observe colour, amount and odour of liquor		
		Apply fetal scalp electrode if fetal heart monitoring is desired continuously		6.3.84 6.30 am
2 Communication				
(i) Inability to cope psychologically with labour due to fear of the unknown, fear of the outcome	No excessive anxiety. Criteria No signs of undue anxiety. States that anxiety is reduced.	Develop a rapport with the client	Throughout labour	
		Allow questions to be asked		
		Give information about i) Each procedure to be performed ii) Maternal and fetal progress iii) Relaxation and breathing exercises iv) Pain relief and availability of analgesia		

Fig. 4.3 (continued)

Potential Problem	Goal	Nursing intervention	Evaluate	Resolved
		Allow a supportive relative to be present in the labour ward		
		Maintain morale		
(ii) Pain. Due to increasing strength of uterine contractions as labour progresses.	Pain controlled to a level acceptable to the client, and consistent with fetal and maternal well-being. Criteria Appropriately relieved of pain yet fully cooperative.	Encourage diversional therapy	Early labour	6.3.84 6.30 am
		Allow client to be mobile		
		Encourage breathing/relaxation exercises		
		Give back massage to relieve back-ache		
		Assess which type and form of analgesia will be most beneficial to client	When necessary	
		Respect the client's own wishes		6.3.84 6.30 am
(iii) Lack of bonding due to: poor maternal interaction with baby. Abnormal baby. Transfer to Special Care Unit	Initiate bonding (Dunn 1981)	Encourage husband to be present at the birth		
		Promote skin-to-skin contact between mother and baby	At birth	
		Promote breast-feeding	In labour ward	6.3.84 6.30 am
3 Breathing (i) Respiratory problems due to emergency anaesthetic intervention	Reduced risk of aspiration. Criteria Stomach known to be empty of food before anaesthetic is induced.	Give only water during labour (Hamilton-Smith 1981)		
		Give Mist. Mag. Tri. 10ml 2 hourly	2 hourly	6.3.84 6.30 am
(ii) Haemorrhage in 3rd stage due to incomplete separation of	Early detection of haemorrhage. Criteria Rising pulse rate,	Give IM Syntocinon 5 Units following delivery of the anterior shoulder		6.3.84 5.20 am

Problem	Goal / Criteria	Nursing action	Timing
placenta, retained products, mucosal tearing	falling B/P, increasing pallor, vaginal bleeding, incomplete placenta.	Check the placenta and membranes	6.3.84 6.30 am
		Examine the vaginal walls for lacerations	
		Observe for bleeding	Following delivery
		Record pulse, temperature and blood pressure	6.3.84 6.30 am
		Seek medical attention if necessary	
4 Eating and Drinking (i) Dehydration due to inadequate fluid intake	Maintain hydration. Criteria Urine output maintained. No soreness of mouth or lips.	Record fluid intake and output	Throughout labour
		Give only water during labour	
		Encourage teeth cleaning	
		Supply mouth wash and glycerine to freshen mouth and lips	
(ii) Ketosis due to increased metabolism, reduced glycogen stores	Prevent ketosis. Criteria No ketosis.	Test each urine specimen for acetone	
		Observe client's breath for acetone	
		Seek medical advice if appropriate	6.3.84 6.30 am
5 Eliminating (i) Full rectum due to constipation	No undue bowel distension or soiling. Criteria Bowel known to be empty prior to labour. Prevention of embarrassment due to soiling.	Give enema if no bowel action for 24 hours (Romney & Gordon 1981)	On admission
		Ensure privacy	
(ii) Urine retention due to pressure on urethra and bladder	No retention of urine. Criteria Able to pass urine normally. No palpable bladder.	Encourage frequent voiding of urine	2 hourly
		Monitor urine output	2 hourly
		Test each specimen for acetone/protein/glucose	
		Using correct aseptic technique, catheterise client if unable to pass urine for over 4–6 hours and bladder palpable (Blannin 1983)	6.3.84 6.30 am

Fig. 4.3 (continued)

Potential Problem	Goal	Nursing intervention	Evaluate	Resolved
6 Personal Cleansing				
(i) Puerperal infection due to bacteria from skin, clothing and air	Reduce the risk of puerperal infection. Criteria Skin is smooth and intact following perineal shave. Skin is clean following a bath.	Perform a perineal shave (Romney 1980)	On admission	
		Encourage client to have a bath	During labour	
		Use correct aseptic techniques when performing these procedures: i) Vaginal examinations ii) Delivery iii) Catheterisations		
		Wear masks when client's vulva is exposed, following rupture of membranes		
		Ensure an adequate supply of sanitary pads		6.3.84 6.30 am
(ii) Perineal lacerations due to tearing or episiotomy during birth of baby	No perineal lacerations. Criteria No undue perineal damage (Needham & Sheriff 1983).	Ensure no grazes or cuts occur during perineal shave	During labour	
		Guard the perineum during delivery		
		Perform episiotomy only in an emergency (Wilkinson 1984). Seek medical assistance to repair tears or episiotomy immediately		
		Give advice regarding perineal care and toilet		6.3.84 6.30 am
(iii) Heavy perspiration due to effect of labouring	Normal standard of hygiene	Encourage client to bathe on admission	On admission	
		Bed bath client following delivery		
		Perform perineal wash-through		
		Ensure a change of nightclothes following delivery		6.3.84 6.30 am

7 Mobilising				
(i) Inability to cope physically with labour, due to exhaustion, ketosis	Enhance maternal well-being. <u>Criteria</u> Ability to cope with contractions.	Develop a rapport with client	Throughout labour	
		Record maternal pulse ⎫	½ hourly	
		Record blood pressure ⎬ Record result on partogram	hourly	
		Record temperature ⎭	4 hourly	
		Ensure adequate rest is achieved		
		Assess progress of labour to determine cervical dilatation, consistency, etc.		
		i) by observation of contractions	½ hourly	
		ii) by vaginal examination.	4 hourly	
(ii) Abnormal uterine action due to hypotonic uterine action or uncoordinated uterine action	Normal progression of uterine action. <u>Criteria</u> No prolonged labour, no ketosis.	Monitor the length, strength and frequency of contractions.	½ hourly	
		Observe for ketosis		
		Seek medical assistance if		
		i) Ketosis present		
		ii) Hypotonic or hypertonic uterine action presents.		6.3.84 6.30 am
(iii) Reduced mobility due to analgesic effects, and the fear of falling	No injuries from falling	Encourage bed rest, or support in a comfortable chair	Following analgesia	
		Do not leave unattended		
		Help onto bedpans as necessary		6.3.84 6.30 am
8 Expressing Sexuality				
(i) Embarrassment/anxiety about intimate procedures	Prevent overembarrassment/anxiety over intimate procedures	Develop 1:1 relationship with the client	Throughout labour	
		Ensure no disruptions during procedures		
		Explain procedures prior to performing them		
		Ensure privacy		
(ii) Lack of privacy in the labour ward	Provide maximum privacy for client	As above		6.3.84 6.30 am

Fig. 4.4 Individualised care plan for Jeanette Turner

Date	Problem (A) actual (P) potential	Goal	Nursing intervention	Evaluation	Resolved
5.3.84	Use along with standard labour care plan/and partogram				
5.3.84 9.00 pm	2 Communicating (a) (A) Anxiety over fetal well-being due to previous microcephalic baby	No excessive anxiety, Criteria Able to talk freely about previous baby. States anxiety is relieved.	Establish a good rapport with Jeanette	9.00 pm until delivered	
			Allow her to discuss previous baby		
			Allow Jeanette the opportunity to ask questions		
			Allow husband's presence in labour ward		
			Discuss and inform parents of fetal behaviour as monitored		6.3.84 6.50 am
			Ensure paediatrician examines baby following delivery	On Post-natal Ward	6.3.84 10.00 am
5.3.84 9.00 pm	3 Breathing (a) (A) Cough related to smoking 10–15 cigarettes daily	No chest infection. Criteria No change in client's normal breathing pattern.	Discourage smoking	Early labour	
			Request doctor examines Jeanette's chest to exclude infection.		5.3.84 10.30 pm
	(b) (P) Inability to use Entonox inhalation analgesia due to respiratory problems related to smoking	To achieve full analgesic effects of Entonox. Criteria Pain relieved to a level consistent with maternal and fetal well-being.	Discourage smoking	Early labour	
			Request doctor examines Jeanette's chest to exclude infection and gain permission to administer Entonox.		5.3.84 10.30 p.m.
	(c) (P) Fetal distress due to nicotine effects	Early detection of fetal distress. Criteria Irregular fetal heart rate Meconium stained liquor.	Monitor fetal heart rate ½ hourly	½ hourly	
			If membranes are ruptured: i) Observe for meconium-stained liquor ii) Apply fetal scalp electrode iii) Obtain continuous ultrasound recording of the fetal heart rate, apply abdominal transducers iv) Notify medical officer		6.3.84 1.20 am 6.3.84 5.30 am

Date/Time	Problem	Goal/Criteria	Nursing action	Timing
5.3.84 9.00 pm	4 Eating and Drinking (a) (A) Heartburn	No heartburn. Criteria Able to take a normal diet without adverse effects.	Give Mist. Mag. Tri. 10 ml 2 hourly	2 hourly
			Modify diet in post-natal period	
			Ensure adequate understanding of food constituents	6.3.84 5.30 am
6.3.84 1.40 am	2 Communication (b) (A) Pain due to strengthening uterine contractions	Pain controlled at a level acceptable to the client consistent with fetal and maternal well-being. Criteria Able to tolerate contractions.	Encourage breathing/relaxation exercises	Throughout labour
			Assess progress of labour by vaginal examination	
			Give most appropriate analgesic	$\frac{1}{2}$ and 3 hours after analgesia
			Assist Jeanette into comfortable position	
	7 Mobilising (a) (P) Potential risk of injury from falling due to analgesic effect	No injuries from falling. Criteria Adequate preventative and protective measures taken.	Advise bedrest, or support in comfortable chair	1.30 am until delivered
			Do not leave unattended	
			Give bed-pans as necessary and assist where necessary	6.3.84 6.50 am
6.3.84 4.20 am	5 Elimination (a) (A) Urine retention due to fetal pressure on urethra	Relief of bladder distension. Criteria Soft abdomen and no discomfort.	Using correct aseptic technique, catheterise client	Following procedure
			Measure and monitor urine output	
			Test urine for ketones, protein and glucose	6.3.84 4.30 am
			Maintain privacy and Jeanette's dignity	

Fig. 4.5 Evaluation of mother's progress

Date/Time	Activity of Living	Evaluation/Progress	Signature
5.3.84
9.00 pm		Client Admitted to Labour Ward in Labour	
	1 Environment	(i) Identiband completed and applied. Case notes checked and correct
(ii) Abdominal palpation performed: Fundus at term
Fetus: Longitudinal lie
Well flexed
Head presenting 3/5 palpable
Left occipito lateral
Fetal heart 138 regular	
	6 Cleansing	(i) Perineal shave performed	
	5 Elimination	(i) No enema at Jeanette's request. Suppositories not required as bowels activated prior to admission
(ii) Specimen of urine obtained: no acetone, protein, or glucose detected	
	7 Mobilising	(i) Maternal observations recorded, all within normal limits. Vaginal examination performed
(ii) Contracting 2:10 lasting 20 seconds	

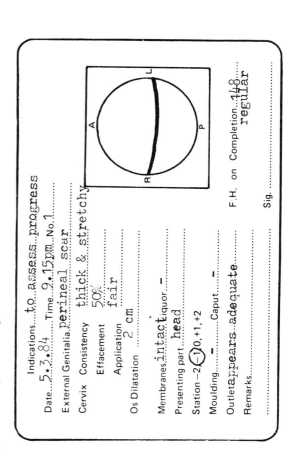

Indications ..to..assess..progress
Date ..5.3.84.... Time .9.15pm.No.1.
External Genitalia.perineal. scar.
Cervix Consistency thick & stretchy
        Effacement   50%
        Application   fair
Os Dilatation ..2 cm

Membranes.intact.Liquor.–
Presenting part .head
Station –2 –1 0,+1,+2
Moulding........ – Caput.... –
Outlet.appears..adequate....
Remarks.......

F.H. on Completion..148......
regular

Sig. ......

Mobility encouraged

Date/Time	Activity	Notes
	4 <u>Eating/Drinking</u>	(a) Mist. Mag. Tri 10 ml given, no heartburn (i) Iced water supplied. Jeanette aware of the reasons why solids are not allowed in labour
	6 <u>Cleansing</u>	(i) Jeanette relaxing in a warm bath
	2 <u>Communicating</u>	(i) Brief explanation of labour given. Jeanette familiar with breathing/relaxing techniques. Husband present
5.3.84 10.30 pm	3 <u>Breathing</u>	(a and b) Jeanette's chest examined by doctor: No signs of chest infection. No indications why Entonox cannot be used (a) Jeanette agrees not to smoke during labour
6.3.84 12 mn	2 <u>Communicating</u>	(a) Jeanette less anxious over fetal well-being, happy that labour is progressing normally. Husband's presence has a supportive and relaxing effect on her
	7 <u>Mobilisation</u>	(i) Jeanette finds walking around comfortable (ii) Contractions increasing in strength 3:10 lasting 40 secs, Jeanette coping well
6.3.84 1.20 am	1 <u>Environment</u>	(iii) Fetal heart 142 regular Liquor ++, slightly blood stained, unoffensive odour Vaginal examination performed

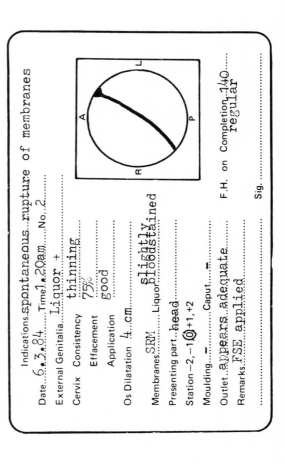

Indications .spontaneous..rupture. .of. .membranes.

Date..6.3.84.....Time.1.20am.....No..2.

External Genitalia... Liquor +

Cervix Consistency thinning

        Effacement 75%

        Application good

Os Dilatation .4..cm

Membranes....SRM....Liquor slightly blood stained

Presenting part..head.

Station −2, −1 ⓪ +1, +2

Moulding... − ....Caput... −

Outlet .appears. .adequate.........F.H. on Completion.140......

Remarks.FSE. .applied.........regular

Sig.....................

Fig. 4.5 (continued)

Date/Time	Activity of Living	Evaluation/Progress	Signature
		Ultrasound transducer and tocotransducer applied to abdomen, recording commenced to monitor fetal heart rate and contractions for $\frac{1}{2}$ hour, to be discontinued if readings within normal range.	
1.40 am	2 Communicating	(b) Contractions increasing to 4:10 lasting 40 seconds. Jeanette tensing and coping less well with the contractions. Requesting Pethidine. IM Pethidine 100 mg, Phenergan 50 mg given.	
	7 Mobilising	(a) Jeanette assisted to bed, feeling drowsy. Nursed well-supported in left lateral position.	
2.15 am	1 Environment	(iii) Fetal heart within range of normal, continuous monitoring discontinued. Recommence $\frac{1}{2}$ hourly observations.	
2.30 am	2 Communicating	(a) Jeanette resting, tolerating contractions well, less tense and anxious	
3.30 am	2 Communicating	(b) Complaining of severe backache. Back rubbed during contractions by husband, with some relief. Entonox inhalational analgesia commenced. Jeanette and husband directed in its use, enabling client to control the input thereby gaining maximum analgesic effect.	
4.00 am	2 Communicating	(a) Jeanette fully in command of Entonox with husband's support. Backache less troublesome.	
4.20 am	5 Elimination	Bladder palpable, Jeanette unable to pass urine normally. Catheterised. 350 ml of urine obtained. No protein, acetone or glucose. States she feels much relieved. Jeanette is experiencing a strong desire to push. Maternal condition stable.	
4.30 am	1 Environment 7 Mobilising	(ii) Fetal condition stable. (i) Vaginal examination to determine progress.	

Indications...assess progress...

Date 6.3.84 Time 4.30am No. 3

External Genitalia heavy show

Cervix Consistency thin

Effacement fully

Application good

Os Dilatation 9 cm

Membranes...R...Liquor bloodstained

Presenting part head

Station −2, −1, 0, (+1) +2

Moulding — Caput —

Outlet appears adequate   F.H. on Completion 150 regular

Remarks fetal scalp electrode in situ   Sig.

2 Communicating   (a) Entonox encouraged
                    (b) Jeanette aware of progress and shows pleasure that the labour is nearly over

Commencement of Second Stage. See Labour Record

5.00 am

Fig. 4.6

PARTOGRAM

Special Points		
Medical	....	-
Surgical	....	-
Obstetric	.1981 Microcephalic/cataracts (died)	
Social	....	

E.D.D. 1.3.84		
Date of Admission to Labour Ward 5.3.84. 9pm		
Onset of Contractions — Time 5.3.84. 6.15pm		
Rupture of Membranes — Time 6.3.84. 1.25am		

Medical Examination		
	Ht 164 cms	
	Wt 89 kgs	
Epidural not wanted by client		

Labour Plan	
Patient's Wishes Husband's presence	
No enema	
Obstetric Plan	

Unit No.	....	
Surname	TURNER	
Forenames	Jeanette Ann	
D. of B.	13.6.61	
Para. 1 (died)	Gravida. 2	

Obstetrician	Mr. Walton	
Anaesthetist	-	
G.P. Hudson	Comm. M/w. Shaw	
Blood Group 0	Rh Factor Positive	Antibodies -

FETAL HEART RATE: 190 180 170 160 150 140 130 120 110 100 90 80 70 60

LIQUOR

URINE
- Vol.
- Ketones
- Prot./Gluc.

LIQUOR	N-O	-	N-O	-	slight blood stained	N-O	C	C cath.	blood stained
Vol.	100				50			350	
Ketones	-	-		-	-			-	
Prot./Gluc.	-		-	-	-		+	+	-
Position of Pt.	walking	sitting	walking	walking	sitting	upright	lt lateral	lt lat	semiprone
Pt's Reaction	relaxed	relaxed	coping	comfortable	tense	coping	coping	backache	fully responsive

DRUGS GIVEN
- Oxytocic
- I.M. Analgesia
- Epidural Analgesia
- Inhalation Analgesia
- Antacids
- Others

Mist. Mag. Tri. 10 ml   Mist. Mag. Tri. 10 ml   Mist. Mag. Tri. 10 ml   1M Pethidine 100 mg   1.40am Phenergan 50 mg   Mist. Mag. Tri. 10 ml   Comm: Entonox   Entonox   Entonox

Midwife's/
Student Midwife's
Signature

Fig. 4.7 Summary of delivery

Midwife's Delivery Notes:

    5.00am   Fully dilated. Presenting part visible. Client fully cooperative
                 Fetal heart rate: 5.05 am 136 regular   5.09 am 130 regular   5.11 am 132 regular   5.14 am 140 regular
                 5.18 am 132 regular
    5.20am   Normal delivery of a live female infant
    5.25am   3rd stage expelled

Maternal Condition after Delivery: Good. Anxiety relieved on seeing and examining baby

Care Given:
    Breast feeding established
    Skin-to-skin contact maintained
    Bed bathed
    Bed-pan offered: unable to pass urine
    Perineal toilet performed

T 37°C P96 B/P 130/60
Uterus firm and central

DELIVERY RECORD

Midwife's Summary of Labour

METHOD of DELIVERY		HAEMORRHAGE	ANALGESIA		PRESENTATION at DELIVERY	
Spontaneous	✓	Third Stage...100...mls.	None		Vertex	✓ Frank Breech
Forceps		Post-Partum.....–.....mls.	**Epidural**	Face		Shoulders
Ventouse		Total....100....mls.	Entonox	✓ Brow		Compound
Section			Trilene	Full Breech		Cord

Placenta and Membranes   Weight. 675   Gms.

How Delivered   controlled cord traction 3 vessels in cord

Comment   placenta healthy, appears complete
2 membranes intact

Oxytocic	Ergometrine		None given	When given	Crowning	After birth of baby	
	Syntocinon	✓		·	Anterior shoulder ✓	After placenta	

Perineum: Intact	✓	Notes on Perineal Repair
1st Degree Tear		
2nd Degree Tear		
3rd Degree Tear		
Episiotomy		
Episiotomy extended		

DURATION OF LABOUR

	LABOUR BEGAN					DURATION		
	DAY	MONTH	YEAR	TIME				
FIRST STAGE	5	3	84	6.15 a.m./p.m.	10 HOURS		45	MINUTES
SECOND STAGE	6	3	84	5.00 a.m./p.m.	HOURS		20	MINUTES
THIRD STAGE	6	3	84	5.20 a.m./p.m.	HOURS		05	MINUTES
				5.25 TOTAL	11 HOURS		10	MINUTES
				I.D.I.	HOURS			MINUTES

Fig. 4.8 Standard care plan for baby

Potential problem	Goal	Nursing intervention	Evaluate	Resolved
1 Safe Environment				
(i) Wrong baby receiving treatment due to mistaken identity	Correct identification and documentation. Criteria No mistakes are made.	Complete two identibands with name, sex and birth date of baby		
		Double check the bands with the parents	Before transfer from labour ward.	6.3.84 6.30 am
		Apply one to baby's wrist and one to ankle		
(ii) Infection of eyes due to bacteria/fungi from vaginal discharge, excretions	No eye infections.	Wipe baby's eyes at birth using sterile swabs	At birth.	6.3.84 6.30 am
2 Communicating				
(i) Abnormality due to fetal maldevelopment and injury	Early detection of abnormality.	Check baby from top to toe, look for obvious abnormalities	Following birth	
		Measure length and head circumference		
		Weigh baby		
	Adequate protective measures taken to prevent injury.	Allow parents to examine their baby		6.3.84 6.30 am
		Request paediatrician examines baby	1st day postnatally.	
3 Breathing				
(i) Respiratory difficulties due to cord compression, drug effects	No respiration difficulties. Initiation of respiration. Criteria Rate and depth of respiration remains within normal limits. Airways clear, colour pink.	Check the cord is not compressed around baby's neck		
		If present, slip over baby's head, or clamp and cut		
		Clear airways using mucus extractor		
		Wipe moisture from baby's nose and mouth		
		Monitor Apgar score (Apgar 1953)	1, 5 & 10 mins.	6.3.84 5.30 am
		If unresponsive, give oxygen via ambubag		
		Seek medical assistance if necessary		

Problem	Goal	Nursing action	Timing	Date/time
(ii) Haemorrhage due to low blood clotting power, deficiency of Vitamin K	No haemorrhage.	Observe for petechial haemorrhage, cephalhaematoma, bruising Securely clamp the cord, observe for oozing Give Konakion 1 mg to all babies at birth	At birth	6.3.84 6.30 am
5 Eliminating (i) Inability to pass urine or meconium due to urethral obstruction, meconium ileus, imperforate anus	Normal bladder/bowel function.	Change napkins when necessary Monitor renal/bowel function Examine baby to exclude imperforate anus	From birth to discharge At birth	6.3.84 6.30 am
6 Body temperature (i) Hypothermia due to poor heat production and loss of heat by evaporation	Retain temperature within range of normal.	Ensure room temperature is 21 to 26.6 C Pre-warm towels and clothes to be worn by baby Use over-head heater to warm baby's cot Dry baby thoroughly following birth Wrap baby, ensuring head is covered in a warmed towel Record rectal temperature (Hill & Shronk 1979) Before transfer from labour ward, supervise breast-feed, or give artificial feed Do not wash baby until body temperature is within normal limits	Prior to the birth 6.3.84 5.30 am Following birth 6.3.84 6.30 am

Fig. 4.9 Condition of Baby at Delivery

CONDITION OF BABY(IES) AT DELIVERY

APGAR SCORING

1 MINUTE SCORE   9

Sign	0	1	2
Heart rate	Absent	Slow (below 100)	Over 100 ✓
Respiratory effort	Absent	Slow irregular	Good Crying ✓
Muscle tone	Limp	Some flexion of extremities	Active Motion ✓
Response to catheter in nostril (tested after oropharynx is clear)	No response	Grimace	Cough or Sneeze ✓
Colour	Pale blue	Body pink Extremities blue ✓	Completely pink

10 MINUTES SCORE   10

Sign	0	1	2
Heart rate	Absent	Slow (below 100)	Over 100 ✓
Respiratory effort	Absent	Slow irregular	Good Crying ✓
Muscle tone	Limp	Some flexion of extremities	Active Motion ✓
Response to catheter in nostril (tested after oropharynx is clear)	No response	Grimace	Cough or Sneeze ✓
Colour	Pale blue	Body pink Extremities blue	Completely pink ✓

INFANT(S) Number born: 1		Sex	Weight	Length	Head circumference
State (A., S.B.) If S.B. (F)resh or (M)acerated		M. F.	Gms.	in cms.	in cms.
Baby 1.	A	F	2950	53.5	34.5
Baby 2.					
Baby 3.					

Delivered by   Senior person present

Method of Resuscitation
Airways cleared using oral suction
Baby cried immediately

Konakion YES/~~NO~~   *Route*   IM

Date/Time	Activity of living	Evaluation/Progress	Signature
16.3.84 Birth 6.30 am	1 Safe Environment	(i) Identibands checked and applied. (ii) Eyes swabbed at birth.	
	2 Communicating	(i) Baby checked from top to toe. No obvious abnormalities detected. Head circumference, length and weight recorded. Parents left alone to examine their baby.	
	3 Breathing	(i) No cord around neck. Airways cleared, cried well. (ii) Holister clamp applied to cord, no oozing.	
	4 Eliminating	(i) Not passed urine or meconium.	
	5 Body Temperature	(ii) Room temperature 22° C. Cot heater on, baby clothes warm. Baby dried thoroughly following birth. Rectal temperature 36.6° C. Good attempt made at breast-feeding.	

References

Association for improvements in maternity services 1983 *Denial of parents' rights in maternity care. London*

Apgar V 1953 A proposal for a new method of evaluation of the newborn infant. *Anaesthesia & Analgesia,* 32: 260

Ball JA 1981 Effects of present patterns of maternity care on the emotional needs of mothers. *Midwives' Chronicle & Nursing Notes,* 94, 1122: 198–202

Blannin J 1983 Catheter guide. *Nursing Times,* Community Outlook, September, 15: 251–263

Carter SL 1980 The nurse educator. In: *Teaching the nursing process.* Nursing Times Publications, London

Central Midwives' Board 1983a *Midwives' Act 1951. Notices concerning a midwife's code of practice.* Central Midwives' Board, London

Central Midwives' Board 1983b *The role of the midwife.* Spottiswoode Ballantyre, London

Dunn DM 1981 Interactions of mothers with their newborns in the first half hour of life. *Journal of Advanced Nursing,* 6: 271–275

Garry MM, Govan ADT, Hodge C & Callender R 1974 *Obstetrics illustrated.* Churchill Livingstone, Edinburgh

Hamilton Smith S 1981 *Nil by mouth.* RCN, London

Hill T & Shronk L 1979 The effect of early parent–infant contact on newborn body temperatures. *Journal of Obstetric & Gynecological Nursing,* September–October: 287–290

Hunt JM & Marks-Maran DJ 1980 *Nursing care plans. The nursing process at work.* HM & M, Aylesbury

Kesby OME 1983 Care in labour—the need for a midwifery policy. *Midwives' Chronicle & Nursing Notes,* 96, 1140: 9

Kratz CR 1979 *The nursing process.* Baillière Tindall, London

Lewis DD 1983 Alcohol and pregnancy outcome. *Midwives' Chronicle & Nursing Notes,* 96, 1157: 420–422

Maslow AM 1970 *Motivation & personality.* Harper & Row, New York

Moir DD 1978 *Pain relief in labour.* Churchill Livingstone, Edinburgh

Needham D & Sheriff J 1983 A survey on tears and episiotomies of the perineum. *Midwives' Chronicle & Nursing Notes,* 96, 1146: 420–422

Nightingale F 1974 *Notes on nursing.* Blackie, London

Parsons T 1952 *The social system.* Tavistock Publications, London

Rogers CR 1951 *Client-centred therapy.* Houghton Mifflin, Boston

Romney ML 1980 Pre-delivery shaving—an unjustified assault? *Journal of Obstetrical Gynaecology,* 1: 269–271

Romney ML & Gordon H 1981 Is your enema really necessary? *British Medical Journal,* 282: 1269–1271

Roper N, Logan WW & Tierney AJ 1980 *The elements of nursing.* Churchill Livingstone, Edinburgh

Roper N, Logan WW & Tierney AJ 1981 *The process of nursing.* Churchill Livingstone, Edinburgh

Roper N, Logan WW & Tierney AJ 1983 *Using a model for nursing.* Churchill Livingstone, Edinburgh

Schifrin B 1979 The rationale for antepartum fetal heart rate monitoring. *Journal of Reproductive Medicine,* 23, 5: 213–221

Spastics Society Hera Unit 1982 *Smoking and pregnancy—a review.* Spastics Society, London

Thompson IE, Melia K & Boyd DM 1983 *Nursing ethics.* Churchill Livingstone, Edinburgh

Webb C 1980 The nursing process—a conflict for nurse teachers? In: *Teaching the nursing process.* Nursing Times Publications, London

Wilkinson V 1984 The use of episiotomy in normal delivery. *Midwives' Chronicle & Nursing Notes,* 97, 1: 106–110

5

Care plan for a woman with squamous cell carcinoma of the cervix, based on King's conceptual framework and theory

Joanne O'Neill ———————————————————

This chapter explores the relevance of Imogene King's (1981) conceptual framework for nurse–patient interaction and her theory of goal attainment with reference to the nursing care of a 32 year old woman undergoing treatment for carcinoma of the cervix. A brief review of the incidence, possible aetiology and treatment of squamous cell carcinoma of the cervix is given and the essential characteristics of King's (1981) conceptual framework and theory are outlined. The conceptual framework and theory are then used to make an assessment of the factors influencing the nurse–patient relationship and goal attainment in the setting described, and this information is then used to devise a plan of care.

Squamous cell carcinoma of the cervix

Incidence and possible aetiology

Each year approximately 4 000 women in England and Wales develop invasive carcinoma of the cervix and over 2 000 women die of the disease (Yule 1984). It is thought that the disease process starts with cellular dysplasia, followed after an indeterminable period by *in situ* changes which usually progress to invasive carcinoma, again after a variable period. Histological changes can be detected as early as cervical dysplasia by a routine screening test, i.e. the cervical smear test. Treatment of both cervical dysplasia and

carcinoma '*in situ*' stops the development of invasive carcinoma and thus, in theory, death from carcinoma of the cervix is entirely preventable. Early invasive carcinoma is itself eminently treatable with at least 80 per cent of women treated for stage I disease (carcinoma confined to the cervix only) remaining disease-free 5 years after treatment. As with all malignancies, the more advanced the disease on first detection the worse the prognosis and only 5–10 per cent of women diagnosed as having stage IV disease (involvement of the bladder and rectum) survive 5 years (Tindall 1984).

Before 1970 the peak age incidence of carcinoma of the cervix was 50 years, but there is now a distinct second peak at about 35 years (Tindall 1984). There is also evidence that the incidence of the disease is increasing (Wolfendale *et al.* 1983, Yule 1984) with the development of a more aggressive form of the disease in younger women (Yule 1984). At one time it was thought that it took approximately 10 years for cervical dysplasia to progress through carcinoma *in situ* to become invasive carcinoma. However, the increasing number of positive smears in women previously known to have had a negative cytological test is beginning to cast doubt on this, and it is felt that recommendations for screening should be changed to include younger women and that screening should be performed more often (Yule 1984).

At present, general practitioners are only paid for screening women who present with symptoms or asymptomatic women who have had more than three pregnancies, or who are over the age of 35 and who have not had a smear within the past five years. Other women may be screened as part of the family planning service or during the routine post-natal examination. Amongst women who are eligible for routine screening there are many who do not make use of the facility, and a large number of women who develop invasive carcinoma of the cervix have never had a cervical smear test. There is no standard national system for following up women with positive cytology, so that it is possible for a woman who has had a positive smear not to be informed of the result of the test and later to go on to develop invasive disease. Such issues are obviously 'politically' sensitive and it is not surprising that women may feel that those with the power have not got their best interest at heart when over 2 000 women each year die from a disease which is preventable. Furthermore, the cost of more intensive screening for the disease would be more than offset by saving on expensive treatment required for invasive disease (Wolfendale *et al.* 1983).

The aetiological agent(s) responsible for squamous cell carcinoma of the cervix remain unknown. Epidemiological studies have shown an association between squamous cell cervical carcinoma and early age of first intercourse (Barron & Richart 1971), early age of first pregnancy (Barron & Richart 1971), high parity (Barron & Richart 1971), multiple marriage (Terris *et al.* 1967), multiple sexual partners (Harris *et al.* 1980) and low socio-economic status (Logan 1954). Other studies have found an association with certain male occupations (Wakefield *et al.* 1973) and promiscuity of the male (Pridan & Lilienfeld 1971).

These epidemiologic observations indicate that cervical neoplasia has many of the attributes of a communicable disease and current research suggests that infection with a virus might play a part. It is thought that certain women may be more likely to develop changes in the cervical epithelium following contact with the virus. Changes in the cervical epithelium occurring during adolescence or while taking oral con-

traceptives may also increase the risk of neoplasia developing (Tindall 1984).

Although it is important for the eradication of the disease that the causative agent is found, the reporting of findings when the picture is still unclear has led to some unfortunate consequences. The public is being told that cancer of the cervix is a venereal disease or an illness women bring on themselves by sexual activity. There is an implicit message that 'a positive smear means you were promiscuous'. The screening that women have campaigned for offers them early detection and treatment at the price of being labelled.

A wider examination of the evidence shows this approach to be inadequate and sexually biased. As long ago as 1971 an Israeli study showed that women could be at risk from their husband's promiscuity. Pridan and Lilienfeld (1971) reported in the Israel Journal of Medical Science the results of a study of carcinoma of the cervix in Jewish women in Israel. Of the women with cancer 37 per cent claimed to have had more than one sexual partner. This is more than the 24 per cent of women with non-malignant disease or the 18 per cent of the general population, but it is nevertheless the minority of patients. When Pridan and Lilienfeld questioned husbands, 74 per cent of those married to women with cancer had had nine or more partners in addition to their wives, compared with 44 per cent of husbands of women with other gynaecological disease and 38 per cent of husbands in the general population. Studies published since then showing a higher rate of positive smears in divorced women have ignored this study and suggested that the women's but not their partners' sexual activity might have been a risk factor.

A study published in 1981 by Buckley *et al.* showed the number of sexual partners reported by husbands to be a significant risk factor. If the husband had 15 or more partners outside marriage, the risk of the wife (who herself had had no other partners) developing cancer of the cervix increased 7–8 times.

Treatment and side-effects

Very early stage carcinoma of the cervix, when there is invasion of less than 5 mm depth, is treated by a simple hysterectomy, or if the disease is more extensive by the more radical Wertheim's hysterectomy. In clinical practice in the UK, radiotherapy is the normal treatment for carcinoma which has spread further than the cervix. Treatment involves both external mega-voltage therapy and intracavity irradiation. In megavoltage therapy, high energy radiation is given to the patient's pelvis, including the tumour, gynaecological organs, bladder, bowel and lymph nodes draining the cervix. Both treatments affect the ovaries and induce pre-mature menopause in pre-menopausal women. In addition, radiation to the bowel causes colicky diarrhoea with mucus production and sometimes severe tenesmus. Dysuria, frequency and haematuria can be caused by the effect of radiation on the bladder. Initially radiotherapy causes an inflammatory reaction, but later this is followed by stenosis and in some cases necrosis. Treatment schedules have to strike a fine balance between giving sufficient irradiation to prevent the spread of the disease and avoiding dosages that will lead to bladder and bowel damage. If the disease spreads the patient may die, and if the bladder and bowel have been severely damaged vesico-vagina or recto-vagina fistulae may de-velop some years after the initial treatment.

Local irradiation of the vagina in intracavity treatment causes stenosis and shortening of the vagina. Immediately after treatment a blood-stained mucous vaginal discharge is common, but after a few weeks the normal mucous secretions of the vagina are no longer produced because the glands are destroyed by the radio-therapy. This has obvious implications for sexual function. The vaginal changes during the normal sexual act have been carefully studied by Masters and Johnson (1966), who have shown that two important phenomena precede the sexual climax. First, there is lubrication of the vagina caused by transudation of mucus through the vaginal wall following a marked dilation of the venous plex-uses which encircle the vaginal barrel. This lubrication is present in post-menopausal women as well as in pre-menopausal women and is therefore unrelated to ovarian function. The other phenomenon is lengthening and expansion

of the upper two-thirds of the vagina as the normal rugae disappear. None of these changes is possible after heavy irradiation because the vaginal wall has lost its elasticity and potential for expansion and there is no source of lubrication. The venous plexus and arteries especially in the upper vagina have been obliterated.

Abitol and Davenport (1974) compared sexual function in 28 women with invasive carcinoma of the cervix treated with radiotherapy with that of 32 women with invasive carcinoma treated by surgery. All women were clinically free of malig-nancy for at least 1 year after treatment was completed, and there was a similar age distri-bution between the two groups. Each patient was interviewed by a gynaecologist and radiothera-pist separately. Information concerning the mode of treatment was withheld from the inter-viewers and the findings of the two interviews were compared. In one case in which major discrepancies were noticed, a third interview was carried out by an independent arbitrator.

The interview covered three areas:

1   Pattern of sexual life prior to the appearance of the disease. The following questions were asked: (i) How frequent was sexual inter-course at that time? (ii) In what percentage of cases was sexual climax reached? (iii) Was the patient interested in sex? (iv) Was there any discomfort or pain associated with coitus?
2   Pattern of sexual life approximately one year after the end of treatment. The same four questions were asked.
3   Other changes in sexual function. If the patient mentioned any noticeable differences between the two previous patterns she was asked to describe what, in her opinion, was the reason for the changes. Table 5.1 gives the changes in frequency of sexual activity following the two modes of therapy.

Among the 28 radiotherapy patients, 12 men-tioned lack of libido and complete or almost complete disappearance of sexual climax. Eleven had marked pain or discomfort during the sexual act. Fifteen had the feeling of a short or narrow

Table 5.1 Changes in frequency of sexual activity following different modes of therapy for carcinoma of the cervix (as reported by Abitol and Davenport 1974)

Type of therapy	No. of patients	Sexual activity				
		Stopped completely	Much less frequently	Minimal change	No change	Improvement
Radiotherapy	28	7	15	3	2	1
Surgery	32	2	0	4	20	6

vagina during coitus. Four had fear of recurrent cancer. Three mentioned that their partner interrupted sexual activity because he no longer found any satisfaction in the act. Ten could not satisfactorily describe their changes.

Among the 32 surgical patients the following changes were noted. Two mentioned lack of libido. One had marked discomfort. Two mentioned short vagina. One interrupted sex because her sexual partner disappeared a few months after the end of her treatment.

Abitol and Davenport had previously documented vaginal and pelvic changes following treatment in the women studied. In the majority of instances when a patient reported sexual dysfunction, she presented a corresponding vaginal change and this was true regardless of the mode of therapy. The authors concluded that adequate radiotherapy for carcinoma cervix produces serious distortion in the anatomy of the vagina in more that 80 per cent of cases, and that in most of these patients sexual dysfunction will occur.

Fear of recurrence of cancer is given by many patients as their reason for sexual abstinence. This is understandable because the accepted view in the medical literature is that cervical cancer has been preceded by a high level of sexual activity. This idea has spread to the lay literature, where cancer of the cervix is linked with promiscuity, and it is possible that some patients imagine that sexual abstinence will prevent recurrence. One may even speculate that in some cases guilt or shame may be involved, since under certain circumstances the cancer could be considered a 'punishment' (Abitol & Davenport 1974).

Reaction to a diagnosis of cancer

The discovery of cancer is typically viewed by the individual who makes such a discovery as a stressful event (Hinton 1973, Peck 1972). It used to be that the debate surrounding the patient's knowledge of the diagnosis fell into two camps— those who said that the patient should know and those who argued that to tell the patient would further increase her existing distress. Now the situation is changing, and the literature suggests that people vary in their need for information on diagnosis and prognosis. Spencer-Jones (1981) and Novack et al. (1979) found that approximately 50 per cent of patients want full information about diagnosis and prognosis while, of the 50 per cent who refused the opportunity for direct discussion, over half indicated that they were aware of their prognosis. Studies have attempted to identify the characteristics of the patient who wishes to be informed. Cassileth et al. (1980) found that younger patients usually wanted more information than older patients, who seemed to prefer a non-participatory role. There is no evidence that prognosis alone is a determinant of whether or not the patient will benefit from knowing the diagnosis.

Within the literature there is evidence of a patient's desire for information relating to treatment and procedures. Even those who do not wish to be given specific details of their diagnosis and prognosis want information about the treatment (Reynolds P et al. 1981, Johnson 1982). Information on the sensory aspects of a procedure is valued (Reynolds S 1981), while the most frequently requested information was about treatment of side-effects and how to prevent or control them (Reynolds S 1981). It has been suggested that depression in cancer patients is linked to feelings of hopelessness and powerlessness over their own destiny (Maguire *et al.* 1980). To give patients knowledge that will help them control side-effects hands back some of the power.

Using nursing theory in clinical practice

My first contact with nursing theory was in an academic context, when different theories were reviewed and evaluated during an MSc programme in nursing. Initially as part of the Master's programme and then later after returning to work as a ward sister, I tested out and applied these theories to try and establish their relevance to the clinical care of the cancer patient. It is my considered opinion that no single theory is sufficient to account for all that takes place in a nursing situation. Different theories are particularly relevant to different stages of the nursing process and practice can be improved by selectively and intelligently combining elements of many different theories. An approach to nursing particularly appropriate to the care of the patient with cancer is as follows:

> Nursing is a process of helping a person *adapt* to the changes illness brings, particularly in relation to the normal *activities of daily living*. The activities of living the patient would usually perform here himself but because of illness or its treatments he lacks the necessary *strength*, *will* or *knowledge*. Nursing *assists* with these activities in such a way as to help the patient to be as independent as possible to carry out *self-care*. The *nurse–patient relationship* is fundamental to these functions, which take place through *nurse–patient interaction*.
>
> (O'Neill 1984)

Elements of many different theories can immediately be recognised in this definition. Theories whose main focus is self-care, stress-adaptation or activities of daily living have been considered in other chapters of this book. This chapter is concerned with the concepts identified in the final section of the definition, i.e. the nurse–patient relationship and nurse–patient interaction, which are fundamental to all stages of the nursing process.

In this second section of the chapter interaction theory is considered in more depth, in particular Imogene King's (1981) conceptual framework for nurse–patient interaction and theory of goal attainment. The theory was used when planning nursing care for a 32 year old woman admitted to hospital for radical radiotherapy for stage II B squamous cell carcinoma of the cervix (carcinoma extending beyond the cervix, involving the parametrium but not as far as the pelvic side wall or lower third of the vagina). The nursing assessment and care plan based on the theory are outlined, followed by an evaluation of the theory and consideration of its implications for education, management and research in nursing.

Interaction

Sundeen *et al.* (1981) state that interaction is a fundamental and inevitable concomitant of nursing, and the steps of the nursing process are implemented through nurse–patient interaction. King (1981) argues that a knowledge of human interaction is essential to nurses, who perform their functions in an interpersonal field. Several nurses have included theoretical frameworks of nurse–patient interaction when writing about the process of nursing. Peplau (1952) proposed that nurse–patient interactions were goal-directed and that nurses and patients grow in the experience. Travelbee (1981) states that there is a purpose in nurse–patient interactions and that the purpose should be known to nurse and patient. Orlando (1961) noted that perception is a key factor in understanding nurse–patient relationships as dynamic and purposeful.

King (1981) defines interaction as 'a process of perception and communication between person and person, represented by verbal and non-verbal behaviours which are goal-directed'. In the person-to-person interaction being considered in this chapter, each individual brings different knowledge, needs, goals, past experiences and perceptions which influence the interactions. King (1981) states that when two individuals come together for a purpose such as a nursing situation, they are each perceiving the other person and the situation, making judgements, taking mental action or making a decision to act. These two individuals react to each other and to the situation. King (1981) argues that reciprocity is an essential characteristic of interaction. When one initiates an interaction with another an action takes place, each person reacts to the other and a reciprocal spiral develops in which individuals continue to interact or withdraw from the situation. King (1981) states that each party has something to give to the other which the other wants or needs, and which may be facilitated by active participation of both individuals in the situation. She also argues that each party has a goal for the interaction. Thus the experience of any interaction is unique to that time and place, and the circumstances and persons involved can never be repeated. King (1981) states that interactions are unidirectional, irreversible, dynamic and have temporal-spatial dimensions. In other words, interactions lead those involved in one particular direction and are influenced by other factors present at that particular time and place. The interaction can never be blotted out, but can only be changed or modified by further interaction. King (1981) feels that nurses and patients respond through interactions to the humanness of each other, to the presence of each other and to the reciprocally contingent (mutually dependent) relationship.

King's (1981) conceptual framework of nurse–patient interaction and theory of goal attainment

The Nursing Theories Conference Group (1980) states that the use and meaning of the terms 'concept' and 'theory' within nursing and other disciplines are often conflicting. This confusion is said to be caused by the frequent use of these terms in a broad, non-defined sense. The Nursing Theories Conference Group defines the terms 'concept', 'conceptual framework', and 'theory' as follows:

Concept – an abstract notion; a vehicle of thought that involves images; an element to develop theories
Conceptual framework – a group of interrelated concepts
Theory – a way of relating concepts through the use of definitions that assists in developing significant interrelationships to describe or clarify approaches to practice

Concepts are grouped together to form a conceptual framework which in turn can be further developed to produce a theory.

Although King (1981) does not define either the term 'concept' or the term 'conceptual framework', her use of both terms is in accordance with the definitions given by the Nursing Theories Conference Group. King states that within her text concepts are used to formulate conceptual frameworks, and concepts and conceptual frameworks are said to be the building blocks for theory development. King's conceptual framework for nursing characterises nursing as taking place within three interacting systems, i.e. personal systems, interpersonal systems and social systems. Nurse–patient interaction takes place in the interpersonal system and King's theory of goal attainment was developed from her conceptual framework for nurse–patient interaction.

Analysis of a theory can give some indication of how useful it might be in practice. In particular, it is necessary to be clear about the assumptions on which the theory is based. For example, it is useful to clarify how the theorist views the roles of the nurse. If the theorist views the nurse as a handmaiden of the doctor, whose only function is to carry out his orders, then anyone using that theory takes on board that assumption; this has obvious implications for practice.

five major elements: a data base, a problem list, a goal list, a plan and progress record; and it was developed from the problem-orientated medical record described by Weed (1969).

The data base is composed of all the information gathered about the patient. This includes the nursing history, the medical history, and reports from social workers and paramedical workers.

From the data base, problems are identified and a problem list is drawn up.

The goal list includes both the goal statement and the process by which the goal will be achieved. It is possible for there to be more than one goal for each problem. For example

Problem 1	Inability to move right arm and leg
Goal 1	Observe and record patient status
Process	a) passive ROM exercises, co-ordinate with physical therapy
	b) Neuro signs q 1 hour and report changes
	c) B/P q 1 hour and report changes
Goal 2	Provide comfort and safety
Process	a) Position in bed and turn q 2 hours and support extremities
	b) Skin care and protection of bony prominences
	c) Mouth care
	d) Call light within easy reach of left hand
	e) Two people to move patient
Goal 3	Discuss nursing care and explain treatments, offer information so patient can participate in care

(King 1981: 170, Fig. 6.3)

NB q = every

It is more usual for the instructions given under 'process' to be included in the plan or intervention section of the nursing record. Indeed it is difficult to ascertain exactly what King (1981) would include under the fourth section of the GONR, i.e. the plan. For this

section she suggests using the Subjective, Objective, Assessment, Plan (SOAP) format described by Weed (1969). But this was originally developed to help describe and evaluate each problem and it is more usually applied to the assessment or evaluation stage of the nursing process.

The fifth element of the GONR is the progress notes. Three types are identified, i.e. narrative notes, flow sheets and the final summary or discharge notes. With regard to narrative notes, King suggests using the SOAP format and giving subjective and objective information about the patient's progress in relation to the problem, and an assessment of the present situation, together with a plan for further action.

Because there appears to be some confusion about what to include in the different sections of the record and because some of the examples given by King are not, strictly speaking, correct (for example to describe 'observe and record patient status' as a goal when it is in fact an instruction) it is difficult to recommend the use of the GONR as described by King. Instead, the more accepted form shown in Figure 5.2, using the headings 'problem', 'goal' and 'intervention' is suggested.

Summary and conclusions

King's (1981) conceptual framework of nurse–patient interaction and theory of goal attainment are most useful to the clinical practitioner if thought of as guides to an approach to care rather than as a set of laws specifying exactly what to do. As previously stated, a comprehensive care plan would require the introduction of elements from other nursing models/theories, e.g. assessmemt of independence in activities of daily living.

The most important points in King's theory are

1   The nurse–patient relationship is fundamental to all stages of the nursing process.
2   Nurse–patient interaction is affected by factors influencing both the nurse and patient, and each interaction is unique.

3   If the nurse and the patient share their perceptions about the problem in order to set mutually acceptable goals, then there is a greater likelihood of the goals being attained than if they had been set by either of the two parties alone.

These elements can be incorporated into the nursing process without the need for specific documentation and they form the basis of an approach to care which is characterised by mutual cooperation between the patient and the nurse.

Fig. 5.2 Care Plan for Elaine Jennings

Problem	Goal	Intervention
1 Unrealistically pessimistic expectations of prognosis due to lack of information	Elaine is able to discuss her prognosis in realistic terms	Arrange for the consultant to discuss with Elaine what is known about the extent of her disease and what in his considered opinion is likely to be her response to treatment. Elaine would like Ian (her boyfriend) to be present. Explore with the ward nurses the factors contributing to their negative attitude towards treatment for cervical cancer. Make sure all staff are aware of the expectations for treatment in Elaine's case.
2 Inability to give 'informed' consent to treatment due to lack of knowledge and incorrect information about possible side-effects	Elaine is knowledgeable about short-term and long-term side-effects. Can relate these to what she knows about possible benefits of treatment (problem 1) and come to an informed decision about her treatment.	Plan and carry out teaching sessions on the following: 1 Short-term side-effects – what to expect, nursing measures and self-care measures designed to minimise side-effects 2 Long-term side-effects, content as above. Elaine would like Ian to be present during these sessions.
3 Feelings of guilt that past behaviour may have caused the disease, due to her limited knowledge of the causes of cervical cancer.	Elaine demonstrates more accurate knowledge about the possible aetiology of cervical cancer. No longer views the disease as 'her fault'.	Explain that the exact cause of cancer of the cervix is unknown, but give information on what is known about risk factors. Point out that there are many factors over which she has no control, and that it is therefore incorrect to blame herself. Elaine does not wish Ian to be present when this is discussed with her, but she said she would like me to see Ian separately.

References

Abitol M & Davenport J 1974 Sexual dysfunction after therapy for cervical carcinoma. *American Journal of Obstetrics and Gynecology*, 119: 181–189

Barron BA & Richart RM 1971 An epidemiologic study of neoplastic disease, based on self-selected sample of 7000 women in Barbados, West Indies. *Cancer*, 27: 978–986

Buckley JD, Dell R, Harris R, Vessey M & Williams P 1981 Case-control study of the husbands of women with dysplasia or carcinoma of the cervix uteri. *Lancet*, 2: 1010–1015

Cassileth B, Zyphis R, Sutton-Smith K & March V 1980 Information and participation preferences among cancer patients. *Annals of Internal Medicine*, 92: 832–836.

Dickoff J, James P & Wiedenback E 1968 Theory in a practice discipline. Part 1 – Practice oriented theory; Part 2 – Practice oriented research. *Nursing Research*, Sept–Oct, 17, 5: 415–435; 17, 6: 545–554

Elkind AK 1980 The nurse as health educator: the prevention and early detection of cancer. *Journal of Advanced Nursing*, 5: 417

Harris R, Brinton L, Cowdell R, Skegg D, Smith P, Vessey M & Doll R 1980 Characteristics of women with dysplasia or carcinoma *in situ* of the cervix uteri. *British Journal of Cancer*, 42: 359–369

Hefferin EA 1979 Health goal setting: patient–nurse collaboration at veterans administration facilities. *Military Medicine*, 144: 814–822

Hinton J 1973 Bearing cancer. *British Journal of Medical Psychology*, 46: 105–113

Johnson J 1982 The effects of a patient education course on persons with a chronic illness. *Cancer Nursing*, April: 117–123

King I 1981 *A Theory for Nursing.* John Wiley and Sons, New York

Logan WPD 1954 Social class variation in mortality. *British Journal of Preventive Social Medicine*, 8: 128–137

Maguire P, Tait A, Broche M, Thomas C &

Sellwood R 1980 The effects of monitoring on the psychiatric morbidity associated with mastectomy. *British Medical Journal*, 281: 1454–1456

Masters WH & Johnson V 1966 *Human sexual response.* Little, Brown and Co, Boston: 293–294

Novack D, Plumer R, Smith R, Ochitill M, Morrow G & Bennett J 1979 Changes in physicians' attitude towards telling the cancer patient. *Journal of the American Medical Association*, 241: 897–900

Nursing Theories Conference Group 1980 *Nursing Theories.* Prentice-Hall, New Jersey

O'Neill J 1984 *The use of nursing records in the evaluation of nursing care.* Unpublished MSc thesis, Manchester University

Orlando I 1961 *The dynamic nurse–patient relationship function, process and principles.* G P Putnam's Sons, New York

Peck A 1972 Emotional reactions to having cancer. *Cancer*, 22: 284–299

Peplau M 1952 *Interpersonal Relations in Nursing.* G P Putnam's Sons, New York

Pridan H & Lilienfeld A 1971 Carcinoma of the cervix in Jewish women in Israel, 1960–67. An epidemiological study. *Israel Journal of Medical Science*, 7: 1465–1470

Reynolds P, Sanson-Fisher R, Poole A, Harker J & Byrne M 1981 Cancer and communication: Information giving in an oncology clinic. *British Medical Journal*, 282: 1449

Reynolds S, Sachs S, Davis J & Hall P 1981 Meeting the information needs of patients on clinical trials: a new approach. *Cancer Nursing*, June: 227–230

Roper N, Logan W & Tierney A 1980 *The Elements of Nursing.* Churchill Livingstone, Edinburgh

Spencer-Jones J 1981 Telling the right patient. *British Medical Journal*, 283: 291–292

Sundeen SJ, Stuart GW, Rankin E & Cohen SP 1981 *Nurse client interaction implementing the nursing process* (2nd edition) Mosby, St Louis

Terris M, Wilson F, Smith H, Sprung E &

Nelson JH 1967 The relationship of coitus to carcinoma of the cervix. *American Journal of Public Health*, **57**: 840–847

Tindall V 1984 Cervical Cancer – 1 Pathology and research. *Nursing Mirror*, **159**, 12: 16–18

Travelbee J 1981 *Interpersonal aspects of nursing*. Davies, Philadelphia

Vachon M, Lyall W & Freeman S 1978 Measurement and management of stress in health professionals working with advanced cancer patients. *Health Education*, 1: 365–375

Wakefield J, Yule R & Smith A 1973 Relation of abnormal cytological smears and carcinoma of the cervix uteri to husband's occupation. *British Medical Journal*, **2**: 142–144

Weed L 1969 *Medical Records, Medical Education, and Patient Care*. Case Western Reserve University Press, Cleveland

Wolfendale MR, King S & Usherwood M 1983 Abnormal cervical smears – are we in for an epidemic? *British Medical Journal*, **287**: 526

Yule R 1984 Cervical cancer – 2 Screening and prevention. *Nursing Mirror*, **159**, 13: 37–39

6

Care plan for an incontinent woman, using Orem's Self-care model

Christine Norton

This chapter describes the designing of a nursing care plan for Mrs Nora Brown, a woman with urinary incontinence, using Orem's (1980) model of nursing. However, initially a little space will be devoted to some background information about the problem of incontinence and to discussing the choice of an appropriate nursing model.

Urinary incontinence

Incontinence of urine is one of the commonest health-care problems among women. The most comprehensive survey to date (Thomas *et al.* 1980) found that 8.5 per cent of women between 15–64 years and 11.6 per cent of those 65 years and over report urinary leakage at least twice per month. Women who have had one or more babies are more likely to be incontinent than the nulliparous. The highest prevalence was found in those women who have had four or more children. Other studies have reported a much higher prevalence of incontinence. Wolin (1969) found that, in a sample of over 4 000 young nulliparous female student nurses, at least one-half reported occasional stress incontinence (leakage upon physical exertion) and 16 per cent reported stress incontinence as a daily occurrence.

The nature of the symptom of incontinence is such that it tends to be concealed by sufferers. Many women seem to expect trouble with bladder control as an inevitable concomitant of childbearing or ageing. As it is so common, many incontinent women know, or know of, a fellow sufferer and so accept the situation without ever seeking help from health-care agencies. Incontinence is also seen as a socially unacceptable symptom producing guilt and embarrassment in those affected. Wolin (1969) found that none of the student nurses in his sample had sought medical attention for incontinence, either because they felt 'ashamed' or because they did not feel that it was abnormal (despite the fact that some had to change their underwear several times each day). Thomas *et al.* (1980) found that only 0.2 per cent of the under-65's and 2.5 per cent of women over 65 years were known to be incontinent by health or social services. Of those with a 'severe' problem, only one in five had sought help. Even those who do seek help may encounter a professional with a negative attitude towards incontinence or without the knowledge and skills to manage the problem effectively.

Continence is a social skill involving far more than merely passing or not passing urine. Modern society has complex, arbitrary rules for acceptable excretion and elimination behaviour. Anyone who does not or cannot comply risks the label 'incontinent'. To be reliably continent necessitates an appreciation of what behaviour constitutes 'continence', the motivation to comply, and the physical ability to do so. It also depends upon an environment geared to the needs and requirements of the individual. Each person must know where the lavatory is and what it is for; be able and want to get there; be able to hold urine and inhibit micturition on the way, and then voluntarily empty the bladder when in the correct position. There are also a host of toilet-related skills and rituals to be performed (cleansing, flushing, handwashing, door locking, removal and replacement of clothing correctly).

Being incontinent has far-reaching implications for the individual. The physical problems of coping with and attempting to contain urinary leakage can be a considerable burden. Development of high-quality incontinence aids has lagged far behind the technical ability and knowledge necessary for the production of reliable products. Sufferers are often unwilling to identify themselves as a potential market and many health authorities attempt to keep expenditure on incontinence aids to a minimum, so there has been little incentive for manufacturers to improve the aids available. The psychological and social implications of incontinence are often as much of a problem as physical coping and are easily overlooked. Norton (1982) found that women expressed the effects of being incontinent mostly in terms of embarrassment and social restriction. Few women were actually physically prevented from activities because of incontinence, but many simply did not want to do things for fear of wetting. Sexual relationships, outings, holidays with the family, shopping, dancing and wearing attractive clothes were commonly avoided or only undertaken in anxious anticipation of an 'accident' occurring. Fear that an unpleasant odour was apparent haunted many women.

Nursing research on incontinence has, with a few notable exceptions, generally been scant. Traditionally nurses have approached the management of incontinence in a piecemeal, unsystematic manner, coping with the immediate effects of soiling rather than seeking long-term solutions to the problem. Reid (1974), investigating the nursing care of ambulant incontinent patients, found that incontinence was 'accepted', indeed not even identified as a 'problem', by the nurses dealing with it. She concluded that 'methods of care for urinary incontinence are bogged down in tradition'. Nurses were reacting purely in an *ad hoc* local fashion with no overall planning or system for care. Reid felt that nurses in fact coped too well in adverse circumstances and unsuitable environments and, by coping,

ensured that the problem never changed. Wells (1980) likewise found that nurses working with the elderly passively accepted incontinence as inevitable. Ramsbottom (1980) describes nursing routines for dealing with incontinence that allowed the patient no participation in care and little dignity or independence. Schwartz (1977) found that both patients and nurses described the other as 'unconcerned' about incontinence, and neither routinely brought up the subject, even while care was being given to remedy soiling. She called this lack of communication 'mutual pretence' that nothing was amiss.

The past decade has witnessed a change in nursing attitudes towards incontinence. A much more positive therapeutic approach is evident, and nursing literature abounds with phrases such as 'the promotion of continence'. As yet this has not been supported by many high-quality studies on what care is most effective, but a problem-solving approach and the attitude that incontinence is something the nurse can do something about are becoming more widespread. At the same time advances in medical diagnosis and treatment have been made. In the UK specialist clinics and nurse specialists (Continence Advisors) are available in some localities (Incontinence Action Group 1983). Much practical advice on assessment, treatment and management is now available (see Norton 1986, for nursing care; Stanton 1984, for medical care).

Nora Brown

Mrs Nora Brown recently consulted her general practitioner (GP) about her incontinence. At consultation she appeared very unwilling to elaborate her symptoms and reluctant to pursue treatment, saying she had only come because her daughter had found out about her incontinence and persuaded her to report it. On physical examination the GP found no obvious physical abnormalities (such as a prolapse) to explain incontinence and diagnosed an unstable bladder (detrusor instability), for which imipramine 25 mg at night was prescribed.

With Mrs Brown's permission, the GP discussed her problem with the district nurse (who was already known to Mrs Brown, having nursed her husband through his terminal illness). Mrs Brown is a 68-year-old widow, formerly very active, recently troubled with arthritis and increasingly socially withdrawn. The GP and nurse together decided that the best course of action was for the nurse to visit Mrs Brown in the privacy of her own home and attempt to gain her confidence in order to assess the situation fully and decide on an overall plan of action.

Choosing an appropriate model

Why should the district nurse use a model in giving care to Mrs Brown? As described above, incontinence has often been approached in a piecemeal fashion. It would be relatively simple for the nurse to visit the lady and give her some incontinence pads and pants, thereby enabling her to cope a little better, while not truly finding out or tackling the real problem. If the nurse is to do more than this she will need to get to know the patient and find out a lot of information about her, because incontinence is often multifactorial in origin and can have extensive ramifications. Reality is a haphazard collection of stimuli of which the nurse must make order and sense. A model will guide the nurse in knowing what information to gather, how to structure contact with the patient and identify appropriate goals; it also facilitates achievement of those goals (McFarlane 1980). A model tells members of a discipline what to look at and speculate about, helps the nurse to focus on what is relevant, gives organisation for thinking, observations and interpretations, and provides general criteria for knowing when a problem has been solved (Fawcett 1984).

Given that a model should help the nurse achieve good patient care, how is an appropriate model to be chosen? McFarlane (1980) believes that, because a model will guide nursing action, it will affect the likely patient outcome. Probably there is no 'right' or 'wrong' model for a given situation; the model merely provides different ways of conceptualising a problem and the

choice, in the end, is subjective and depends on the value system of the nurse. As long as a model is reasonably sound, any will do and the nurse should seek one congruent with her beliefs (Fawcett 1984).

Incontinence is such a common nursing problem that a nursing model which could not guide care for an incontinent woman would not be very useful as a general theory of nursing. Any of the well-known models could be used in helping Mrs Brown and several would fit well. Roy's (1980) concept of adaptation to tension (from within or from the environment) would guide the nurse in examining Mrs Brown's four subsystems (physiological needs, self-concept, role function, and interdependence). It would also help the nurse to identify points of tension, in order to restore the balance by manipulating the relationship between environmental stimuli and Mrs Brown's own adaptation level. Johnson (1980) sees the nurse as helping the individual maintain behaviour within societal norms and achieve equilibrium within her eight subsystems. Continence would fit well into this behavioural model. Riehl's (1980) interaction model is developed from self-concept theory and sees responses as based on the meanings attached to actions. Mrs Brown's reluctance to discuss her problem and her social withdrawal suggest problems with self-concept and the nurse will need to examine the meaning of the symptom to her. An 'activities of daily living' model (e.g. Roper 1976) views eliminating as one of the basic essentials of human activity. Each of these models would approach the problem of incontinence from a different yet valid perspective.

However, for a patient living at home for whom it is reasonable to anticipate eventual rehabilitation to complete independence from nursing care, Orem's (1980) model seems most appropriate.

Elements of Orem's nursing model (Orem 1980)

The district nurse decides to use Orem's model in assessing and managing Mrs Brown's incontinence. Orem's central concept and goal is that of *self-care*. Orem sees nursing as a helping service, with foundations that are biological, behavioural and social. She states, 'nursing is action performed by nurses for the benefit of others'. However, this means collaboration with the patient, not merely doing things to her. Orem values the individual's own ultimate responsibility for self-care, with the patient moving towards self-sufficiency in self-care wherever possible (as opposed to the tendency to medicalise everyday life). The nurse–patient relationship is essentially complementary, their behaviours and actions combining to achieve the patient's self-care. Obviously not all people require nursing—how does the nurse identify those who do? Orem believes the need for nursing arises out of the individual's (or her carer's) inability to maintain self-care – 'nursing has as its special concern the individual's need for self-care action and the provision and management of it on a continuous basis in order to sustain life and health, recover from disease or injury, and cope with their effects.'

Although some of the component tasks involved in nursing may be simple, it is essentially complicated for one person (the nurse) to do something for another that the patient cannot do, must not do, or prefers not to do. The nurse must conceptualise the whole situation and fit tasks into a larger overall design for self-care. The model expresses a commitment to the patient as a whole and tends to emphasise health rather than ill-health, a positive preventive focus. The theory gives a basis for organising patient information and gives a focus to the nurse's endeavours.

Orem advocates the use of the Nursing Process and describes the nursing role as within a multidisciplinary team approach to health care. She stresses that a nursing diagnosis is not a substitute for medical care and that the roles of the various professions are complementary, hence the importance of effective communication between all involved professionals to ensure all are seeking compatible results for the patient. These professionals share four operations of practice – diagnosis (what is, and why); prescription (what should be/what can be); treatment (putting into operation prescribed courses of action); and management (coordinating a dynamic integrated system of care).

Terminology

Some of the terminology used by Orem may be unfamiliar. This should not be allowed to deter the reader, as the terms express important ideas succintly. The following summarises the key terms and should be referred to when reading the rest of this chapter.

Self-care is a learned behaviour that purposely regulates human structural integrity, functioning and human development. Every person requires self-care; when it is not maintained illness, disease or death will occur. It is the practical response to the experienced demand to attend to one's self.

Self-care requisites are the kinds of actions necessary to achieve self-care. Orem distinguishes three categories – universal, developmental and health-deviation self-care requisites (or needs).

Therapeutic self-care demand is the totality of actions to be performed to meet self-care requisites. A system of self-care is 'therapeutic' to the degree to which it (1) supports life processes and promotes normal functioning, (2) maintains normal growth, development and maturation, (3) prevents, controls or cures disease processes or injuries, (4) prevents or compensates for disability.

Agent is the person taking action.

Self-care agent is therefore the person taking action to achieve self-care. This may be the individual for herself, a family member for a dependant (**dependant-care agent**) or a nurse acting for a patient.

Self-care agency is the ability to engage in self-care.

A **nursing system** is the product of nursing practice, formed when nurses prescribe, design and provide nursing.

Diagnosis

Orem views determining whether individuals or groups have needs or requirements that nurses can legitimately meet as an essential nursing action. The nurse then proceeds to make a more detailed investigation of nursing requirements. 'The art of nursing includes making a comprehensive determination of the reasons why people can be helped through nursing.' The nurse must investigate and understand what self-care requisites exist and judge what can and should be done—what is the nature of the demand and what action will constitute a therapeutic response? The nurse cannot know the self-care demand of an individual unless it is calculated – ideally the patient eventually will be able to calculate her own demand.

Orem is very specific about the nature of nursing diagnosis. Each universal self-care requisite should be particularised together with any existing, emerging or projected developmental or health-deviation requisites. Having determined that Mrs Brown actually needs nursing, the nurse will examine her self-care demands and abilities in detail and look for any deficit which can be remedied by nursing action (Fig. 6.2). Orem believes that the nurse requires highly developed specialised skills to calculate the therapeutic self-care demands of patients. To do this she will both observe the patient and communicate with the patient and her family and the responsible physician to determine their perspectives of the problem. The nurse will need a complete picture of Mrs Brown from a nursing care perspective, an image of her as a person. Specifically, the nurse will gather information of personal details, cultural, social and educational factors, characteristic behaviours and anything else which is felt to be relevant (Fig. 6.1).

Nurses obtain, sort out and interpret the meaning of many types of information. Orem advises being selective and gathering only sufficient information to answer five basic questions:

Fig. 6.1 Personal Profile

Name	Nora BROWN Age 68 years
Marital Status	Widow (husband died following a cerebrovascular accident 3 years ago).
Occupation	Retired, previously taught secondary school English.
Residence	Lives alone in own semi-detached house, bathroom and lavatory upstairs
Family	Has two married daughters. One lives 10 mins walk away and visits 2–3 times per week. The other lives 20 miles away – Mrs Brown used to spend alternate weekends with her but has recently stopped (because of bed-wetting). Has three grandchildren.
Developmental state	Mrs Brown appears a mature, intelligent adult. Has adapted poorly to retirement, bereavement and advancing age. Has lost interest and motivation for activities in and out of the home.
General health state	Mrs Brown says her health has, all her life, been excellent until the past two years when her arthritis first became troublesome. Now has some restriction of movement because of pain and stiffness. Appears somewhat depressed and apathetic, lacks former energy and vitality.
Health perspective	Mrs Brown sees health as 'given'—something that happens to you over which the individual has little control. Appears passive and accepting of own arthritis and incontinence – 'it's just old age'. Incontinence causes her shame and she tries to hide it – she was most upset when her daughter found out. Her husband was incontinent for the last months of his life – she fears she may be at the end of her life also. Is not complying with GP's advice on arthritis as she knows it is 'incurable'.
Social activities	Was formerly active in Townswomen's Guild and a bridge club. Has a small circle of friends, neighbours and former colleagues. Virtually all social contacts have lapsed recently. No longer goes to church.

1 What is the patient's current and future therapeutic self-care demand?
2 What is the patient's deficit in self-care agency to meet the therapeutic self-care demand?
3 What is the nature of and reasons for this deficit?
4 Should the patient refrain from self-care or protect her abilities?
5 What is the patient's potential for future self-care?

Information is gathered for a purpose and must be useful. The use of survey lists is recommended in commonly-recurring situations. The theory provides a basis for organising the otherwise potentially confusing mass of patient information.

Figure 6.2 shows the diagnostic information gathered by the nurse about Mrs Brown. This was not all obtained at an initial visit; the picture developed over three visits and after consultation with the GP and Mrs Brown's daughter (with the patient's prior permission). As Orem states, it often takes a long time for the nurse to understand what nursing is required. Where self-care deficits exist the nurse must find out why (e.g. does the patient have a deficit of skills, knowledge, motivation, or a limited repertoire of behaviour for cultural or developmental reasons?). The individual's potential for present and future self-care will determine what the nurse will have to do and the feasibility of actions.

The nurse should identify the interrelationship of requisites. Mrs Brown has an unstable bladder, causing symptoms of frequency, urgency, urge incontinence and nocturnal enuresis. This is much exacerbated by her poor mobility and manual dexterity, which mean that she cannot get to or onto the lavatory quickly. Her home is poorly adapted to her physical needs. As she does not wish to see herself as 'disabled', she has not sought appropriate aids to self-toileting. Her poor diet, low fluid intake and immobility are likely to be the cause of her constipation, which in turn exacerbates bladder problems. Her poor social and interpersonal functioning and low morale and self-esteem mean that she lacks motivation to remedy the situation. She is unwilling to socialise because of incontinence, but her loneliness merely reinforces her lethargy (as may the constipation). As she has not sought help the incontinence is poorly controlled – considerable soiling of clothing and furniture is apparent, as is a definite unpleasant odour in the house. This has added to her low self-esteem.

This assessment will be continuing and will need updating over time as Mrs Brown's self-care demand and abilities progress.

Prescription: nursing system design

Following diagnosis, the nurse must evaluate and interpret the information gathered and organise it into a meaningful order. Orem's emphasis is on the preventive nature of health care – as primary, secondary or tertiary prevention (i.e. prevent, cure, or contain and cope). The individual's therapeutic self-care demand is essentially a prescription for continuous self-care action through which identified self-care requisites can be met with stipulated degrees of effectiveness. The nurse must be most specific in planning care.

The complementary role of nurse and patient is important here. The nurse does not simply design a plan for care but negotiates with the patient an appropriate system that will be both therapeutic and acceptable to the patient. The model assumes that the patient is willing to adopt certain roles and desires to achieve self-care. In the long term the nurse aims to restore the patient to a state of balance between self-care demands and abilities.

A total design for self-care action should be formulated, taking into account the interrelatedness of problems and ensuring that courses of action designed to meet one requisite do not interfere with the achievement of other goals. The approach should not be piecemeal and the care plan should be quite specific about time, place, environmental conditions and the equipment and supplies required for the production of the nursing system. The activities of the patient, nurse and significant others are specified, as are the care measures, resources and any coordinating activities necessary. The care plan should give the 'who, what, when and where' of methods for reaching goals. Once again, this will need to be modified over time as abilities and demands change.

The general goals of a nursing system Orem sees as three-fold

1 The patient's therapeutic self-care is accomplished
2 Nursing actions help move the patient toward responsible action in self-care (increased independence or adaption to inabilities)
3 The patient's family becomes increasingly competent in caring

The plan should help keep actions in line with goals and coordinate the activities of nurse, patient and others. The nurse should be constantly aware of what the patient is experiencing and feeling. Ideally the nurse's role is that of assisting the patient in making enquiries, decisions and plans wherever this is possible and prudent. Always the person being helped should understand what needs to be done, what to expect and what to report.

Orem describes five methods of nursing assistance: acting for another; giving guidance or physical and psychological support; creating a developmental environment; and teaching another. When designing a nursing system the nurse has the choice of three helping systems: a wholly compensatory system (when the patient is unable or must not engage in self-care activity); a partly compensatory system (both nurse and patient perform some self-care measures); and a supportive-educative system (where the patient needs help in relation to decision-making, behaviour control or acquisition of knowledge or skills). The nurse negotiates with the patient to devise the most appropriate system.

Figure 6.3 shows the initial care plan devised for Mrs Brown. It is a mixture of the partly compensatory and supportive-educative modes of help. This would necessarily be modified over time as her self-care abilities changed and, if goals were being achieved, movement would gradually be towards a purely supportive-educative system.

Evaluation

Orem sees evaluation as an integral part of a nursing system. Once the system is designed and planned, the nurse must put it into operation and manage it. Evaluation should check what was done against what was specified to be done; collect evidence to describe the results of care and use this evidence to evaluate the results achieved against the results specified in the nursing system design. The model gives the criterion of self-care as a basis for evaluation of effectiveness of nursing care—has the therapeutic self-care demand of the patient been met?

Conclusion

Orem's model of nursing enabled the District Nurse to conduct a systematic assessment of Mrs Brown's problems. This revealed a set of inter-related problems each of which, if remedied, would help in enabling her to achieve continence. The (fairly) extensive assessment enabled the nurse to pick up problems which, had they remained unidentified, might have worked against the success of therapy for the unstable bladder (i.e. imipramine and bladder training). So, although using Orem's model required time and effort during initial contact with the patient, it possibly saved time in the long run. Also, by enabling more comprehensive nursing care, it ensured that care was given to the *whole* individual, rather than just the problem for which she was referred. By picking up some problems relatively early (e.g. constipation or immobility) the nurse may have been able to prevent them becoming troublesome enough to warrant a nursing referral in their own right.

If the comprehensive assessment is done properly, it should enable easy identification of key problems for the care plan. This means that the care plan from which the nurse and patient actually work can be a realistic length, concentrating only upon what is relevant.

By using Orem's model, the nurse is guided towards enabling the patient to be self-caring as soon as possible. This ensures that patients are not simply taken on to the nurses' caseload and remain there *ad infinitum*. This makes it a particularly appropriate model for community care, where the nurse must constantly try to rehabilitate people to independence to make way for new referrals.

Some problems may be encountered in using Orem's model. For some patients the optimistic view of the patient's role and own contribution to health care may be unrealistic. A few of the terms used are imprecisely defined, such as 'therapeutic', 'sufficient', and 'normalcy'. The nurse has to use professional judgement as to the value

of these for each patient (which may not always coincide with the views of the patient, or indeed those of other members of the health care team). Some of the parameters used are difficult to measure accurately (for example self-care agency – it is easier to see what is not being accomplished than why). Clinical research is contributing to the resolution of some of these problems and developing instruments for measuring outcomes (see Fawcett 1984, for an annotated bibliography of research using Orem's model).

In conclusion, Orem's model of nursing provided a good framework for the District Nurse's assessment and care planning in the case of Mrs. Nora Brown.

Fig. 6.2 Assessment

Self-care requisites	Therapeutic self-care demand	Current self-care abilities	Self-care deficit	Future potential for self-care
(a) Universal				
1 Maintain sufficient intake of air	Breathe normally unassisted.	Self-caring	None	Self-caring
2 Maintain sufficient intake of water	Drink a variety of fluids, as desired, at least 1.5–2 litres/24 h.	Unwilling to drink for fear of incontinence. Constantly thirsty.	Knowledge deficit – does not realise fluid restriction is counter-therapeutic. Motivation deficit – cannot be bothered to make a cup of tea.	If Mrs Brown understands importance of adequate fluid intake and getting a drink can be made easier, she should become motivated to adequate self-care.
3 Maintain sufficient intake of food	Prepare and eat a nutritious well-balanced diet.	Is not eating well, either quality or quantity.	Knowledge deficit – need for high-fibre diet for the sedentary person. Motivation deficit – cannot be bothered to cook for one. Skills deficit – difficult to get shopping and to prepare food because of arthritis.	Unlikely to be completely self-caring unless arthritis improves – will need to accept some help with shopping and food preparation. Should learn to plan own well-balanced diet.
4 Care associated with eliminative processes	(a) Bring about and maintain conditions necessary for regulation.	Has lost ability to inhibit and delay micturition reliably until lavatory is reached – has episodes of urgency, frequency, urge incontinence, nocturia and nocturnal enuresis.	Skills deficit, probably due to unstable bladder. Motivation deficit – has had so many 'accidents' sometimes does not bother trying to get to the lavatory.	Will depend upon response to imipramine and bladder training. If motivated to cooperate should become continent and resume normal micturition pattern within 6–12 weeks.
		Is grossly constipated.	Is not taking enough fibre, fluid or exercise to assist bowel function.	Should be able to become self-caring.

Self-care requisite	Goal	Assessment	Deficit	Expected outcome
(b) Manage the process of elimination and disposal of excreta.		Has difficulty getting to and onto the lavatory because of arthritis and stairs. Often has urge incontinence while removing clothing. Does not wake in time at night. Has difficulty cleaning up after leakage.	Skills deficit – poor mobility and dexterity. Environmental deficit – poor adaptation of house to needs. Resource deficit – does not have appropriate aids or clothing.	With appropriate aids and adaptations, should be able to self-toilet.
(c) Provide subsequent hygienic care of body.		Arthritis in hands prevents effective cleaning of genitalia. Unable to bath herself.	Skills deficit – cannot manage cleaning. Knowledge deficit – unaware of safe transfer methods.	Should achieve effective use of lavatory paper with aids. May need nursing help for a bath.
(d) Care for the environment to maintain sanitary conditions.		Is not always effective in attempts – odour apparent.	Skills deficit – manual dexterity poor. Resource deficit – has no effective pads to protect.	Appropriate aids should prevent soiling.
5 Maintain a balance between activity and rest	An activity level which stimulates interest and maximises mobility. Enough rest for recuperation.	Immobile and inactive by day. Sleep broken at night by nocturia.	Functional deficit – mobility is painful. Skills deficit – cannot inhibit bladder. Motivation deficit – has given up many activities.	Should overcome frustration and lethargy by re-focus of activities to within range of physical abilities. Sleep should improve if bladder becomes more stable.
6 Maintain a balance between solitude and social interaction	Activity level avoids loneliness yet maintains autonomy and independence.	Is lonely yet unwilling to socialise. Feels unable to fulfill roles of mother and grandmother.	Role-model deficit – has image that she cannot live up to of capable, energetic person. Support deficit – does not wish to discuss problems with family or ask for help because of embarrassment.	It may be possible to persuade Mrs Brown to accept more dependent-care from family. Unclear how difficult it will be to resume former friends and pastimes.
7 Prevent hazards to life, well-being and functioning	Be alert to potential hazards and take appropriate action to prevent, remove or control.	Good	None	Good

Fig. 6.2 (continued)

Self-care requisites	Therapeutic self-care demand	Current self-care abilities	Self-care deficit	Future potential for self-care
8 Promotion of normalcy	Realistic self-concept	Feels herself to be abnormal – incontinent and disabled.	Knowledge deficit – does not realise incontinence is common and curable. Support and motivation deficits.	Should be capable of adjusting self-concept and resuming normal lifestyle.
(b) Developmental Maintain living conditions that promote maturation. Prevent or mitigate conditions that affect human development.	Successful transition to retirement, widowhood and advancing age and role as grandmother. Accept some degree of dependence.	Seems to be coping poorly with newer roles.	Knowledge deficit – unaware of many positive features of role. Support deficit – does not use available support optimally.	With counselling, guidance and support, may achieve maturation and growth.
(c) Health-deviation 1 Seek and secure appropriate medical assistance	Consult GP about arthritis and incontinence.	Has, somewhat reluctantly, sought appropriate help.	None	May need encouragement to maintain appropriate behaviour.
2 Be aware of and attend to effects of pathological conditions	Needs to know about therapeutic care for arthritis.	Passive, negative attitude to care.	Knowledge deficit. Motivation deficit.	If understands importance of maintaining residual function and preventing immobility and stiffness, should be self-caring with guidance and encouragement.
3 Effectively carry out medically prescribed measures	Consistently take prescribed drugs for arthritis and bladder. Follow exercise programme.	Unreliable use of medication. Failure to exercise.	Motivation deficit. Knowledge deficit – does not fully understand purpose of medication or exercise.	Good, if becomes motivated.

4 Be aware of and attend to side-effects of medical care	Look for and report side-effects.	Unaware of possible side-effects	Knowledge deficit	Good
5 Modify self-concept to accept self as being in a particular state of health and in need of health care	Accept and actively participate in medical and nursing care offered.	Reticent in accepting need for help.	Self-concept deficit. Motivation deficit.	It should be possible to enable Mrs Brown enough autonomy and independence in care to allow her to accept help.
6 Learn to live with effects of pathological conditions in a life-style that promotes continued personal development	Live with arthritis (and incontinence if it proves intractable) while resuming a more satisfying life-style.	Not coping well.	Attitude and motivation deficit.	Mrs Brown will need a lot of support and guidance to adapt her life successfully.

Fig. 6.3 Care plan

Self-care goal	General helping methods	Specific care actions (DN = District Nurse; NB = Nora Brown)
1 Controls urgency of micturition and avoids urge incontinence. Voids urine at 3–4 hourly intervals and 0–1 times at night within 3 months.	Teach and support	DN to teach general bladder physiology and mechanism of urge incontinence. Method of bladder training (explain keeping chart and practise delaying micturition). Review chart for progress and advice every 4 days initially. Teach role of medication. DN support – attempt to motivate NB to carry out bladder training and take imipramine as prescribed. NB to record all episodes of micturition and incontinence on chart provided. DN to liaise with GP in reviewing medication after one month.
2 Gets to and onto lavatory quickly and effectively.	Provide developmental environment	DN to request an occupational therapy home assessment to select appropriate aids (e.g. stair rail, grab rails around lavatory, raised seat). NB's daughter to help her modify clothing and purchase some that is easier to manage when toileting. DN to order a bedside commode for night use.
3 Manages elimination, hygiene and any incontinence so that any soiling or odour is avoided.	Provide developmental environment. Teach	DN to teach effective methods of cleansing and transfer. DN to assit NB with weekly bath, attempting to encourage her to safe independence within one month. Occupational therapist to provide any aids necessary for this. DN to order appropriate pads and pants for NB (review supply in one month to check appropriateness of type and amount supplied). NB's daughter to help with washing of bedlinen.
4 Relieve current faecal impaction and prevent future constipation. Aim to restore former habit of one bowel motion on alternate days.	Act for. Guide and teach	DN to give NB a course of three disposable enemas (one daily) and then re-assess impaction. DN to teach causes and prevention of constipation and guide NB in choice of appropriate diet, fluid and exercise level. NB should recognise when laxatives are appropriate. Daughter to give assistance at weekly shopping expeditions and to bring fresh fruit and vegetables on regular visits.

5 Increases fluid intake to at least 1.5 litres/24 h	Teach and guide	DN to teach importance of sufficient fluid intake and how to calculate intake. Guide NB in selecting appropriate fluids and times for drinks. Occupational therapist to assess whether aids would make this easier.
6 Resumes a more 'normal' and satisfying life-style so that NB feels satisfied with her role.	Guide and support	DN to discuss self-concept and changing roles with NB. Assess need for more formal counselling after one month of contact. Encourage NB to take up former activities, possibly with help (e.g. could a friend give her a lift to meetings?). Ask friends in for a drink rather than a meal if cannot cook. Is likely to feel more able to socialise once incontinence is improved and controlled – discuss this with NB as bladder training progresses.
7 Follows prescribed care for arthritis.	Teach, guide and support	DN to teach the pathology of arthritis and the importance of maintaining function and control of symptoms. Guide NB in selecting an appropriately graded plan of activity and rest such that her activity gradually increases to maximum attainable. Support NB's efforts to comply with exercise programme and medication prescribed. DN to liaise with GP and report NB's progress.

References

Fawcett J 1984 *Analysis and evaluation of conceptual models of nursing.* F A Davis Company, Philadelphia

Incontinence Action Group 1983 *Action on incontinence.* King's Fund Centre, London

Johnson DE 1980 The behavioural system model for nursing. In: Riehl JP & Roy C (Eds) *Conceptual Models for Nursing Practice.* Appleton-Century-Crofts, New York

McFarlane EA 1980 Nursing theory: the comparison of four theoretical proposals. *Journal of Advanced Nursing,* **5**: 3–19

Norton CS 1982 The effects of urinary incontinence in women. *International Rehabilitation Medicine,* **4**: 9–14

Norton CS 1986 *Nursing for continence.* Beaconsfield Publishers, Beaconsfield

Orem DE 1980 *Nursing: concepts of practice* (2nd edition) McGraw-Hill, New York

Ramsbottom FJ 1980 *Toileting and changing elderly patients in hospital.* Department of Geriatric Medicine, University of Birmingham

Reid EA 1974 *Incontinence and nursing practice.* M Phil Thesis, University of Edinburgh

Riehl JP 1980 The Riehl interaction model. In: Riehl JP & Roy C (Eds) *Conceptual models for nursing practice.* Appleton-Century-Crofts, New York

Roper N 1976 *Clinical experience in nurse education.* Churchill Livingstone, Edinburgh

Roy C 1980 The Roy adaptation model. In: Riehl JP & Roy C (Eds) *Conceptual models for nursing practice.* Appleton-Century-Crofts, New York

Schwartz DR 1977 Personal point of view – a report of seventeen elderly patients with a persistent problem of urinary incontinence. *Health Bulletin,* **35**: 197–204

Stanton SL (Ed) 1984 *Clinical gynecologic Urology.* CV Mosby Company, St Louis

Thomas TM, Plymat KR, Blannin JP & Meade TW 1980 Prevalence of urinary incontinence. *British Medical Journal,* **281**: 1243–1245

Wells T 1980 *Problems in geriatric nursing care.* Churchill Livingstone, Edinburgh

Wolin LH 1969 Stress incontinence in young, healthy nulliparous female subjects. *Journal of Urology,* **101**: 545–549

7

Care plan for a woman with an ectopic pregnancy, based on Roper's Activities of Living model

Susan Cowen

This chapter presents a nursing care plan for a patient admitted to the casualty department with a ruptured ectopic pregnancy. The care plan focuses on the period prior to emergency surgery, and is based on the Roper, Logan and Tierney Activities of Living Model (1980). The chapter begins with a definition of ectopic pregnancy and a discussion of related medical and nursing research, and its nursing implications. This is followed by the introduction of a patient, a discussion of the models available and reasons for choosing the Roper model in planning care. An outline of Roper's model is given, followed by an assessment of its teaching and management implications and finally a critique of the model.

The complete pre-operative care plan is shown, but a post-operative plan of care is not included because of limited space.

Ectopic pregnancy

The word ectopic comes from the Greek 'ektopos' which means 'out of place'. An ectopic pregnancy is a pregnancy which implants outside the uterine cavity; it may also be called an extra-uterine pregnancy.

The commonest site for an ectopic pregnancy is in one of the Fallopian tubes (MacKay *et al.* 1983), 95 per cent being tubal, as Figure 7.1 shows. About half of these tubal implantations are found in the ampullary portion of the Fallopian tube (40–55 per cent). Although implantation may take place in the abdominal cavity, ovary, or cervix, each of these sites is rare (3–5 per cent). Most cases of abdominal implantation are secondary to ruptured tubal gestation. The co-existence of an intra-uterine pregnancy

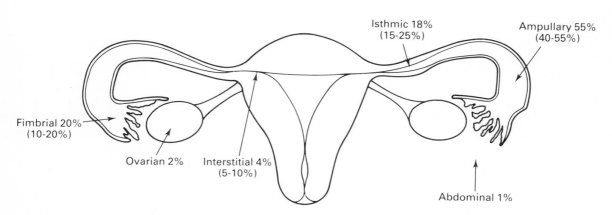

Fig. 7.1 Sites for ectopic pregnancy

with an ectopic pregnancy, although rare, is not unknown.

The outcome of an ectopic pregnancy in pathological terms will vary according to the site of implantation. If the ovum embeds in the narrow isthmus of the Fallopian tube it may burrow deeply and eventually erode the wall, causing tubal rupture and internal haemorrhage. A ruptured tubal pregnancy is a gynaecological emergency, as the patient may die rapidly from hypovolaemic shock. This is the most dramatic outcome of ectopic pregnancy, and it is perhaps for this reason that ectopic pregnancy is a frequent topic in nursing examinations! Sudden death, however, is not the commonest outcome and ectopic pregnancy most often presents as a chronic illness. Because of the non-specific signs and symptoms, it may easily be confused with conditions such as appendicitis. Patel (1985), in a five year study of ectopic pregnancies, revealed that only 18 per cent (12 of 67) of patients presented with the classical acute picture. Most patients studied presented with a subacute form of ectopic pregnancy (55), and a correct diagnosis was not made until at least 24 hours after admission in 29 of these cases.

Research into ectopic pregnancy

Most research on ectopic pregnancy is carried out by doctors and looks at incidence, causes, and effects on future fertility. Ectopic pregnancy is a major factor in maternal mortality. Although the overall maternal mortality rate has declined, the number of deaths due to ectopic pregnancy has not (Beral 1975). Thus ectopic pregnancy is the cause of an increasing proportion of maternal deaths. In fact, the incidence of ectopic pregnancy in the USA, Britain, Finland and Sweden has increased substantially since the late 1950s, with a noticeable increase and doubling of incidence in the 1970s (Beral 1975). Weinstein *et al.* (1983) have called this rise in incidence 'the new surgical epidemic'. Johns (1984) has stressed that ectopic pregnancy is a serious health problem and therefore a serious nursing problem.

Many reasons have been put forward to account for this increase in incidence. Pelvic inflammatory disease is thought to be a major cause of ectopic pregnancy (Westrom 1975), but other possible causes include intra-uterine contraceptive devices (Westrom *et al.* 1981), the progesterone only pill and induced abortion (Beral 1975), previous abdominal and tubal surgery and a previous ectopic pregnancy (Chaukin 1982). The incidence seems to increase with age, particularly in the 25–34 age group (Beral 1975).

Psychological effects of ectopic pregnancy

The implications of these research findings for nurses involved in gynaecological and well woman care are many. Nurses working in these areas will not only be involved with the physical care of patients but also with the psychological care, social influences and health education. Although no specific research has been published to date on the psychological effects of ectopic pregnancy, a woman with a ruptured ectopic pregnancy is likely to suffer psychological trauma on four accounts:

1   the emergency nature of the admission and subsequent surgery
2   the loss of the pregnancy
3   altered self-concept
4   the effect on future fertility

The first of these, the emergency nature of the admission and subsequent surgery, are both anxiety-provoking. Patients having routine surgery are known to experience anxiety both before and after their operation (Wilson-Barnett 1979), and many studies have demonstrated the effectiveness of psychological preparation for surgery (Ridgeway & Mathews 1982). Some have shown the importance of information-giving in reducing post-operative complications (Hayward 1975, Boore 1975). In emergency surgery the problems are exacerbated by the limited time available for giving information and the condition of the patient. One may therefore hypothesize that a patient may not only face surgery with high anxiety levels but may also develop more post-operative complications.

Grief is usually interpreted as both a reaction to loss and a process of realisation (Speck 1978). Grief, and also anger and confusion, may therefore be reactions experienced by women who have lost a pregnancy. Oakley *et al.* (1984) suggest that in the case of an ectopic pregnancy the grief may be more difficult to come to terms with because the woman will be unable to see the pregnancy and may find it difficult to believe that it was there. The process of realisation may therefore be delayed. Guilt may accompany the grief, particularly if the woman has had a termination of pregnancy in the past, and this pregnancy is a wanted pregnancy. Depression may occur and be difficult to overcome. Oakley *et al.* (1984) have described how partners play a very important part in supporting women through their process of grieving after miscarriage. Self-help groups may also help a woman to come to terms with her loss. Although no specific group exists for women who have suffered an ectopic pregnancy, groups such as the Miscarriage Association may be of value. Webb (1984) describes the expansion in the USA of the nurse's role in women's health care, particularly in setting up self-help groups. Perhaps British nurses can learn something from their American counterparts.

Altered self-concept, the third cause of psychological trauma, may occur for several reasons. The effect of surgery, the scar, the loss of a Fallopian tube and sometimes an ovary, may all cause the woman to feel she is incomplete, mutilated or not a 'proper' woman any longer. This feeling of loss may affect her relationship with her partner and family, and she may feel that she has failed her partner in not having a successful pregnancy. All these can result in depression which may manifest itself in several ways, such as loss of interest in appearance, in sex and in social activities. Expert counselling including both the woman and her partner will be required in order to reassure the woman that she is a worthwhile person in herself for her many positive qualities, and that this incident has not changed her value to herself and to others.

The effect on future fertility may be a great concern, particularly if the woman is in her later twenties and childless. Surgery is life-saving, but the type and extent of surgery which should be performed remains controversial (Patel 1985). Patients with ectopic pregnancy have their fertility impaired by between 33 and 60 per cent (Anon 1976). Nagamani (1984) suggests that the uterine pregnancy rate for a woman with a previous ectopic pregnancy and pelvic inflammatory disease is poor (19 per cent). These patients share a high recurrence rate (27 per cent). Oakley *et al.* (1984) do not paint such a gloomy picture, suggesting that the overall risk of a second ectopic pregnancy is 10 per cent. The decision about whether to try to become pregnant again must be made by the woman and her partner after receiving professional advice.

Choosing an appropriate model

A nursing model is a logical representation of what nursing is or ought to be. As this book demonstrates, there are several types of nursing models which can be used in planning patient care. The common or shared feature of all these models is that patient care in each is personalised and individualised.

The patient chosen for this care plan was a 27 year old married woman, Susan Jones, who was admitted via the hospital casualty department in a collapsed state due to a ruptured ectopic pregnancy. She was accompanied by her husband, John, who looked very distressed and anxious. The Jones' had been married for two years and this was a planned pregnancy.

Susan had had a termination of pregnancy at the age of 19 and after this had developed severe salpingitis. She had been using the combined pill as her method of contraception and had discontinued its use three months prior to admission.

Susan worked as a hairdresser and John was a

self-employed plumber. They lived in a council maisonette in the East end of London. John and Susan were both brought up in the 'East end' and Susan's parents live nearby.

In choosing a model the life-threatening nature of the patient's condition and the need for speedy care must be considered to be of importance. A full assessment of the patient's normal routines was not initially possible, and it is suggested that a second assessment should be completed after surgery. An Activities of Living (AL) model seemed appropriate. On admission Susan's ALs were severely disrupted and she was totally dependent on medical and nursing staff, particularly for her physical and physiological needs, but this was a relatively short crisis period. After surgery, once her body's homeostasis was re-established, she was quickly nursed back to almost complete physical independence in the ALs but still needed psychological support. Before discharge she had achieved total independence in physical ALs but psychologically still needed help.

The majority of nursing models originate from North America and have been influenced by work within the field of human sciences. There are, therefore, some similarities of content between the models. McFarlane (1980) attempted to compare the models of King, Rogers, Orem and Roy. She suggested that they all were concerned with nursing as a discipline assisting a man or woman to reach their optimum health level. How this was achieved differed from model to model. 'While King spoke of meeting man's basic needs, Rogers saw the nurse's role as promoting the interaction between man and his environment. The nurse, according to Orem, seeks to influence man's development in achieving an optimal level of self-care whereas Roy viewed nursing as promoting man's adaptive abilities' (McFarlane 1980).

In Susan's case it was felt that the holistic (life process) model (Rogers 1970) was inappropriate. Rogers' model stresses that the patient's response is necessary in order for the goal to be reached. At the time of admission Susan was unable to be involved significantly in goal-setting and had definite physical priorities for care. The life-threatening problems had to be dealt with first

and there was insufficient time for mutuality of goal-setting between Susan and the nurse. Orem's self-care model (Orem 1971) seemed inappropriate, as its main assumption is that the individual wishes to be self-caring. The nurse is seen as a possible self-care agent, but the main goal is patient self-care. On admission Susan was not capable of deciding one way or the other whether she wished to self-care. King's general systems model (King 1968) stresses a mutuality of relationship between the nurse and patient in realising a goal. This may not have been possible in Susan's case and so the model was considered inappropriate. Roy's adaptation model (Roy 1970) could have been used. The nurse in this case is seen as the supporter and promoter of adaptation who manipulates focal, contextual and residual stimuli. This model is particularly appropriate for psychological care (see Chapter 8) and in this area might have proved more useful.

Roper's (AL) model was used because it relates to activities with which every person is familiar, namely living activities. The concepts introduced in the Roper model are relatively simple to understand and, unlike the American models, it does not use elaborate terminology. Both these factors mean it can be introduced at the beginning of nurse training. Furthermore Roper's model was devised by a British nurse educator and has been applied practically with success in the British health care setting. Therefore the model was considered best suited to the clinical teaching context in which it was devised to assist nurse learners.

Elements of Roper's nursing model

This model was first proposed by Roper (1976) in a research monograph and further developed by Roper, Logan and Tierney (1980) in *The Elements of Nursing*. It is a model of nursing based on a model of living. People are regarded as individuals involved in a process of living throughout their lifespan, from conception to death. Each individual performs certain activities during the living process, some of which are essential for the maintenance of human life. Dying is also included and is seen as the final act of living. Roper (1976) identified 16 activities of daily living (ADLs) but Roper, Logan and Tierney (1980) amended the list to 12 activities of living (ALs), and the revised list will be used in this chapter.

The ALs do not remain static but are continually changing, being affected by physical, psychological, cultural and socio-economic factors as the individual pursues the process of living. Furthermore some ALs may have priority over others. This concept of priority is not new, and Abraham Maslow (cited in Child 1981) suggested in his hierarchy of human needs that they may be placed in order of priority. Roper *et al.* (1980) also describe three broad patterns of behaviour affecting the ALs, namely preventing, comforting and seeking activities.

The model also includes a dependence/independence continuum, as there may be periods in the lifespan when the individual is unable to perform the ALs independently. When this happens, problems may occur. Examples given of dependency periods are childhood, old age or during illness. Roper *et al.* (1980) also cite additional factors which may decrease the individual's independence, namely disability and disturbed physiology, pathological and degenerative tissue changes, accident, infection and the physical, psychological and social environment. The main goal during the process of living is to attain self-fulfilment and maximum independence in each activity of living and therefore to remain problem-free. Good health is an essential element in the achievement of this goal.

One must now ask the questions, 'What is the relevance of Roper's model of living for nursing?' and 'How can it be used as a model of nursing?'. A definition of nursing is perhaps required. Roper (1976) defines nursing as follows:

> Within the context of a health care system and in a variety of conditions, nursing is helping a person towards his personal independent role of the continuum of each activity of daily living, helping him to remain there, helping him to cope with any

movement towards the dependent pole or poles and because man is finite, helping him to die with dignity.

The links between the process of living, as depicted in Roper's model, and nursing can be seen by looking at this definition. The model is useful for identifying nursing activities and grouping them together, thus enabling nursing to be structured. Giving structure to nursing care links well with the nursing process which has been described as 'a systematic problem-solving approach to care' (Binnie *et al.* 1984). Roper *et al.* suggest that people who need nursing have some sort of health problem, be it actual or potential, which affects their ability to carry out ALs, and they have applied the nursing process to their model of nursing in *Learning to Use the Process of Nursing* (1981) and also in *Using a Model for Nursing* (1983).

A nursing model will only be used successfully if it is acceptable to practising nurses, and for this to occur the knowledge base of the nurse must be sound. During initial assessment of the patient the nurse needs to apply knowledge of body structure and function, as well as communication skills, in order to obtain accurate information from the patient. Physical, psychological and social changes will result in real and potential problems related to the ALs. The position of the individual on the dependence/independence continuum also has to be decided, together with the priority of each problem identified after initial assessment; when problems, both real and potential, have been identified, goals may be stated and nursing care planned. Implementation of care may then take place, followed by evaluation of its effectiveness and reassessment of the problems.

Before Roper's model could be used to plan nursing care for Susan Jones, several points needed clarification. Roper, during assessment, focuses on normal routines and what a patient can or cannot do independently. Webb (personal communication 1985) suggests it is also necessary for the nurse to consider how the ALs are affected by the patient's current health status/illness/disability. This is essential in order to

Fig. 7.2 Pre-operative care plan for Mrs Susan Jones

Activities of living	Date and time	Assessment	Problems (A) actual (P) potential	Goal
Maintaining a safe environment	2.3.85 10 pm	Vital signs: Blood pressure 70/40 Pulse 40, weak Vaginal loss: slight, red Skin: cold, clammy	(A) Hypovolaemic shock due to ruptured ectopic pregnancy	Correction of shock, vital signs stable
		Susan complains of severe, spasmodic, stabbing pain in left side of lower abdomen, which started at 6 pm.	(A) Pain	Pain control: Susan says she has no pain, points to 'no pain' end of painometer
		Doctor has decided that urgent surgical intervention is required	Preparation for theatre. (P) Error of Susan's identity or operation	Ensure Susan delivered to theatre with correct documentation
Breathing	2.3.85 10 pm	Vital signs: Respiratory rate 40, depth shallow, rhythm regular, panting. Colour of skin and nailbeds: blue	(P) Respiratory arrest secondary to hypovolaemic shock. (P) Airway obstruction	Susan's respiratory function maintained within normal limits, potential problems avoided
Communicating	2.3.85 10 pm	Susan looks pale, eyes staring, says she is afraid. Husband says he is also anxious. Appears drowsy on admission	(A) Anxiety due to pain, bleeding, emergency admission and impending surgery. (P) Loss of consciousness due to shock	Less anxiety: Susan says she feels more calm. Facial expression more relaxed. Neurological state stable, Susan more responsive
Eating and Drinking	2.3.85 10.30 pm	Time of consumption of last food 7.30 pm, last drink 8 pm. Vomited once (100 ml), partly digested food. Complaining of nausea	Full stomach (P) Inhalation of vomit during anaesthesia (P) Dehydration	Susan's stomach emptied and potential problem resolved. Moist mouth, normal skin tone and urine output, no thirst. Susan says she has no nausea
Eliminating	2.3.85 10 pm	Bladder empty – last passed urine at 4 pm	(P) Renal shutdown due to hypovolaemic shock	Maintain sufficient urine output to excrete waste products, i.e. 300 ml per 24 hr minimum.
		Bowel full – last opened 2 days ago	(P) Peritonitis or bowel obstruction	Detect any complications immediately they occur. No bowel perforation

Nursing intervention	Evaluation/progress	Rationale
Management of IV fluid replacement. Record intake and output. Record PV loss – colour, amount. Monitor vital signs $\frac{1}{4}$ hourly – inform doctor if pulse exceeds 160 or BP falls below 70/40. Observe skin colour. Lie flat. Do not tip bed. Remain with Susan.*	Hypovolaemic shock stabilised at 12 min	*Elevating the foot of the bed is not recommended, because any free fluid/blood in the abdominal cavity may irritate the diaphragm, causing respiratory arrest.
Observe for signs of discomfort, restlessness, guarding. Administer prescribed analgesia and monitor its effectiveness using painometer*. Position Susan confortably.	Pain relief achieved by 11 pm	*Ensure analgesic does not cause severe hypotension
Identify Susan with wristband. Doctor to obtain consent for operation. Nurse accompanies Susan to theatre with notes	Susan safely identified and prepared for theatre at 12.30 am on 3.3.85	
Monitor and record respiratory rate, depth and rhythm $\frac{1}{2}$ hourly. Maintain airway – nurse in semiprone position. Administer oxygen as prescribed, observe colour. Inform doctor of blood loss	Satisfactory respiratory rate (18) on transfer to theatre at 12.30 am on 3.3.85	
Stay with Susan at all times. Explain all procedures and give information. Give support and explanations to husband.	Susan appeared less anxious on transfer to theatre at 12.30 am on 3.3.85.	
Assess neurological state $\frac{1}{4}$ hourly. Record vital signs, response to commands, pupil reactions and size, response to painful stimuli. Report any change immediately to doctor	Stable neurological state achieved at 12 mn	
Nothing by mouth from admission. Pass nasogastric tube and aspirate gastric contents. Record amount of aspirate.	Prepared safely for anaesthesia at 12.15 am.	
Give anti-emetics by injection as prescribed. Record vomit on fluid balance chart. Offer mouthwashes as required	Nausea controlled by 12 mn. Mouth moist, Susan says she is not thirsty. Urine output – see Eliminating	
Record urine output $\frac{1}{2}$ hourly	100 ml of urine passed between 10 pm and transfer to theatre at 12.30 am.	
Do not give bowel preparation*	No signs of perforation of bowel on transfer to theatre	*Stimulating the bowel of a patient with obstruction may cause perforation and death

Fig. 7.2 (continued)

Activities of living	Date and time	Assessment	Problems (A) actual (P) potential	Goal
Personal cleansing and dressing	2.3.85 11.30 pm	Requires urgent preparation for theatre	(P) Post-operative wound infection due to contamination by bacteria from skin/clothing	No infection
Controlling body temperature	2.3.85 10 pm	Admission base temperature 38.5°C	(A) Pyrexia – ? infection ?peritonitis	Temperature 37°C within 2 hours
Mobilising	2.3.85 10 pm	Unable to move on admission due to pain	(P) Pressures sores (P) Deep vein thrombosis (A) Pain	No pressure sores. No deep vein thrombosis. Susan says she has no pain
Expressing sexuality	2.3.85 10.30 pm	Tearful. Husband says this was a wanted pregnancy	(A) Loss of pregnancy and effect on body image, relationship with husband and future fertility	Susan will voice her feelings to husband and nurse and show her emotions
Dying	2.3.85 10.30 pm	Tearful and says she is afraid. Husband also says he is anxious	(P) Death of patient (A) Loss of potential baby.	Susan will express her fears and grief

define the problem(s). Susan was in need of emergency care and required surgical intervention to restore physiological homeostasis. The initial nursing assessment on admission could not be fully completed because of the patient's inability to communicate and her need for speedy care. Priority problems were identified by the nursing staff (Fig. 7.2), breathing and safety needs being more essential than sleeping. Some information was obtained from Susan's husband, but it was felt that a second assessment would be needed after surgery. Information regarding

Susan's normal routines would then be obtained. Roper *et al.* (1983) suggest that assessment should be continuous, and so this fits in well with their model of nursing.

Because dealing with Susan's physiological needs was a priority, there was a danger of ignoring her psychological needs. Nursing staff were only able to give a brief explanation to Susan of what she might expect, and information-giving in this case was limited compared with that given to a patient admitted for planned surgery. It was felt that psychological

Nursing intervention	Evaluation/progress	Rationale
Give wash, shave or use depilatory cream to remove pubic hair if pulse below 100, BP above 100/60, and Susan's pain controlled at level of no pain on painometer. *Put on theatre gown.	To be evaluated post-operatively	* If in a severe state of shock Susan should be disturbed as little as possible and transferred quickly to theatre without being washed or shaved
Monitor temperature $\frac{1}{4}$ hourly. Reduce temperature by use of fan and tepid sponging if it rises above 40°C. Treat infection by administering antibiotics as prescribed. Give preventive care to reduce intra-operative infection risk – see Personal Cleansing and Dressing.	Temperature 36.4°C at 12 mn	
Give prescribed analgesia. Monitor effect with painometer. Turn hourly.	Pain free by 11 pm, no signs of pressure sores or deep vein thrombosis on transfer to theatre	
Clear explanation of operation to be given by nurse. Explain clearly nature of operation, position of lower addominal scar. Allow Susan to express her fears. * Information about future fertility should not be given until post-operatively. Arrange for counselling post-operatively.	Fears expressed and Susan less tearful at time of transfer to theatre	* Until surgeon has isolated the site of the ectopic pregnancy a prognosis about future fertility is impossible to give
Allow Susan to voice fears. Maintain life by correcting problems and achieving homeostasis. Explain loss of fetus. Arrange for post-operative counselling.	See Expressing Sexuality	

support after surgery would be a nursing care priority.

If Susan's operation had been planned, a standard nursing care plan could have been used for pre-operative preparation for anaesthetic and surgery. An additional plan showing her specific problems could then have been completed. In Susan's case it was considered important to complete fully the pre-operative care plan, as the care was implemented immediately by the casualty department nursing staff. Her care and the plan would then be transferred to the theatre nursing staff and post-operatively to the ward nurses. This short period of time in the casualty department enabled the use of Roper's model in planning care to be illustrated completely. Disruption of Susan's normal routines of sleeping and working and playing had occurred, but it was felt more appropriate to include them on the post-operative ward care plan than on the casualty department care plan. A post-operative care plan is not shown because of limited space.

Teaching and management implications

The value of a nursing model depends on how easily it can be implemented in the practical nursing situation. There is some controversy about whether this is easily achieved. In order for a model to be applied successfully, three requirements must be fulfilled. Firstly, the model must be fully understood and accepted by both trained staff and nurse learners. Secondly, the model must be suitable for the particular health-care setting in which it is being used. Thirdly, all paper work must be lucid and minimal. If these three criteria are fulfilled, the model should find acceptability and therefore be both useful and successful.

The two main groups of people on which the successful use of the model depends are nurse teachers and nurse managers. The former ensure that the model used is suited to the particular nursing environment and the background knowledge of the nurses concerned, while the latter see that it is implemented on the 'shop floor'. Roper's model is unusual in that it has been, and is being, used on the 'shop floor'. The implications of Roper's model for nurse teachers and nurse managers will be discussed separately.

For the nurse teacher, Roper's model has the inestimable advantage of being easily taught—and understood. Roper's model is in line with some basic tenets of educational psychology (Child 1981). For example, the model enables the nurse learner to perceive patient care in a structured way. Perception is an essential part of the learning process and, as the gestalt (German for pattern or form) school of psychology suggests, we should enforce structure to promote perception because individuals see patterns as wholes. New nursing recruits using the nursing process for the first time often flounder. They ask, 'What are we assessing?' and generally become confused. Roper's model promotes structure and therefore simplifies the learning process. Because Roper's model focuses on activities of living and normal, observable routines it is easily conceptualised. It can be introduced early in the nurse training programme and used to plan patient care. Indeed, schools of nursing could use Roper's model as a framework to structure the content of the curriculum. The starting point for such a curriculum could be health, healthy people and their activities of living, and health care systems, moving on later to ill-health and illness. Relevant anatomy and physiology, sociology, psychology and communication skills could be introduced at appropriate points along the way.

As a clinical teacher, I have found Roper's model very useful for junior learners because it helps them to bridge the gap between what is taught in the classroom and the real-life patient on the ward. The activities of living can be used as a check-list, but in doing so must be viewed broadly. For example, surgical patients may have their safety disrupted by a problem such as haemorrhage. The nurse learner will identify this as a problem and the teacher may then guide the learner by linking knowledge of the signs and symptoms of hypovolaemic shock to the patient and the care plan. Diagrams are useful visual aids to help link the learner's knowledge of anatomy and physiology to the patient's condition.

Implementation of research findings may be achieved using an activities of living framework. An example of this might be the use of Hayward's painometer (Hayward 1975) as a means of measuring whether a goal has been achieved.

For nurse managers the implications of Roper's model are rather different. It has been mentioned that all members of the ward team are important if the model is to be successfully implemented. For trained staff to be comfortable with a model and to be able to use it with the nursing process, they too must have a good knowledge base. Study sessions may be arranged in collaboration with the unit manager, using the expertise of such people as staff development tutors and the nursing process co-ordinator, in order to update the knowledge of trained staff.

For both trained staff and learners, use of a model should help in questioning and escaping from the rigidity which has been a feature of our profession for so long. Models should make both the teaching and learning of nursing more exciting. Because Roper's model is adaptable, ward tutorials can be organised using care plans based on it. Evaluation of care and the updating of care plans using the model can also be used as another teaching opportunity during ward reporting sessions. This encourages trained staff and learners to question in a positive way the care they are implementing.

Health education is an important aspect of nursing, and Roper's model is particularly useful in teaching patients. Initial assessment of the patient's normal routines offers an ideal opportunity for the nurse to explain to the patient what to expect. Research has shown that blanket reassurance to reduce anxiety is not helpful (Ridgeway & Mathews 1982). Factual information about what to expect is more useful. The factual information may be verbal or may be provided in booklet form for the patient to read later. When the nurse is explaining, for example, where surgery is to be carried out, diagrams may be used as visual aids. Webb and Wilson-Barnett (1983), following their research with hysterectomy patients, suggest that it is not enough to explain a topic once and think the information has been retained. Nursing staff should incorporate information-giving at each stage of patient contact, thus promoting retention and thereby reducing anxiety.

Nurse managers and nurse teachers need to work together in looking at systems of management for the delivery of nursing care. The essential component of a nursing model and indeed of the whole process of nursing is individualised patient care. If ward management is arranged on a task allocation basis the model will not work. Nurse managers also need to consider other professional aspects, such as accountability and its inevitable legal implications. The UKCC code of professional conduct (1984) stresses that all registered nurses must be accountable for their practice. Two of the points in the code of practice are particularly relevant for nurse managers where the nursing process is being used. One stresses the promotion and safe-guarding of the interests and well-being of patients. The other is that no action or omission on the part of

the nurse should affect or be detrimental to the safety of the patient. If care is planned by nurse learners using a nursing model, the trained staff are ultimately accountable for patient care. Thus care plans should be checked and ideally be signed as correct by trained staff. This re-emphasises the point that a model and its documentation must be acceptable to and understood by all members of the ward team. More experienced learners should also be allowed to choose which model they think is most suitable for their patients. The commonest complaint about the nursing process by those using it is that the paper work is endless. Webb's quotation (1984) is apt: 'On the eighth day God created the nursing process and nobody rested!'

To conclude, using a model of nursing with the nursing process gives structure to care planning. This should make the process easier and quicker, and should ultimately improve patient care. If practical problems are overcome, models may even in the long term be cost-effective by reducing patient dependency and thus the length of a patient's stay in hospital.

Critique of the model in use

Evaluation of the care plan devised by using Roper's model was possible before Susan Jones went to theatre. In this relatively short space of time, several apparent problems with the usage of the model became evident. One of these was the inappropriateness of the model for an emergency situation. To focus on normal routines of the patient, related to activities of living, seemed pointless as the patient was already in an abnormal state and had grossly disordered activities of living. The position of the patient on the dependence/independence continuum was more relevant, but problems arose when trying to plot the patient's position on the continuum. An accurate method of doing this could not be agreed upon and therefore the exercise appeared valueless in the absence of precise criteria for measuring dependence/independence. Indeed, a full assessment as suggested by Roper was not possible in view of the need for emergency care.

However, a second assessment was completed post-operatively and, as Roper *et al.* (1983) suggest that assessment should be a continuous process, this was in line with their ideas.

The ability of Roper's model to help plan psychological care was questionable. Deciding exactly where psychological problems fit into the framework of the model may be difficult. The danger of concentrating on physical problems to the exclusion of psychological problems was an area of concern. Perhaps Roy's Adaptation Model (1970) might have been more suitable for planning psychological care post-operatively because of its focus on psychosocial aspects of adaptation.

The amount of paper work the model involved led to criticism. Roper *et al.* (1980) have suggested that the activities of living can be used as an 'aide memoire' and therefore do not have to be written down. This would reduce the size of the care plan. A rationale need not constitute part of the plan, particularly if clear explanation of the reasons for carrying out a particular procedure are given by the trained staff on the ward. However, rationales are invaluable for teaching purposes. Evaluation could have taken place in the 'Kardex', thus reducing the size of the care plan. If this was done, a small review column would be required on the care plan.

As discussed in the section on teaching and management implications, Roper's model is easily conceptualised, particularly by junior learners. In my experience some senior learners become bored with the model. They regard it as too simplistic an approach to planning care. Perhaps when this happens it is time to introduce other models into the curriculum and allow more senior learners to decide which suits their patients best. On the other hand, it is hard to envisage it being practical to have several different models in use concurrently on a ward.

In conclusion, Roper's model has undergone modification since it was first suggested in 1970. This is because it has been used practically and it is open to change. This is supported by Logan who says, 'Models too are artefacts. They are meant to grow, adapt, change and be discarded, if no longer useful' (cited in RCN Nursing Standard 1985). This is a statement we should all consider when using nursing models!

Acknowledgements

I would like to thank Mr A Doherty, Librarian, Mrs J Easterbrook, Head of Department (Staff Development), and Miss C Harper, Administrator, all of the Nightingale School at St Thomas' Hospital, for their help and advice. Churchill Livingstone have granted permission for the use of Figure 7.2 from *Using a Model for Nursing* (1983) by N Roper, W W Logan and A J Tierney. I am also grateful to Miss Hunter for typing and retyping the chapter and to Dr C Webb for being such a supportive editor. Finally, my thanks go to Martin for his continued patience, support and encouragement.

References

Aggleton P & Chalmers H   1984   Models and theories – 1 – Defining the terms. *Nursing Times*, 5th September: 24–28

Aggleton P & Chalmers H   1985 Models and theories–6–Roper's activities of living model. *Nursing Times*, 13th February: 59–61

Anon   1976   Tubal pregnancy and surgery (Editorial). *British Medical Journal*, 1: 607–608

Beral V   1975   An epidemiological study of recent trends in ectopic pregnancy. *British Journal of Obstetrics*, 82: 775–782

Binnie A, Bond S, Law G, Lowe K, Pearson A, Roberts R, Tierney A & Vaughan B   1984   *A systematic approach to nursing care an introduction*. Open University, Milton Keynes

Boore JRP   1975   *Prescription for recovery*. Royal College of Nursing Research Series RCN, London

Chaukin W   1982   The rise in ectopic pregnancy – exploration of possible reasons. *International Journal of Gynaecology and Obstetrics*, 20: 341–350

Child D 1981 *Psychology and the teacher* (3rd edition) Holt, Rinehart and Winston, London

Hayward J 1975 *Information-a prescription against pain.* RCN, London

Hewitt S R 1976 Ectopic Pregnancy. *Nursing Times,* 26th August: 1308–1310

Johns J L 1984 Ectopic pregnancy. *Nurse Practitioner,* June: 17–22

King I M 1968 A conceptual frame of reference for nursing. *Nursing Research,* 17: 27–31

MacKay E V, Beischer N A, Cox I W, & Wood C 1983 *Illustrated textbook of gynaecology,* Saunders, Sydney

McFarlane E A 1980 Nursing Theory: The comparison of four theoretical proposals. *Journal of Advanced Nursing,* 5: 3–19

Nash T G 1974 Extra-uterine pregnancy. *Nursing Times,* 17th October: 1623–1624

Nagamani M, London S & St Amand P 1984 Factors influencing fertility after ectopic pregnancy. *American Journal of Obstetrics and Gynecology,* 1st July: 533–535

Nursing Standard 1985 Report of a two day conference on 'Models of Nursing', No. 394, 25th April: 2 (RCN, London)

Oakley A, McPherson A & Roberts H 1984 *Ectopic pregnancy in miscarriage.* Fontana paperbacks, London

Orem DE 1971 *Nursing: concepts of practice.* McGraw-Hill, New York

Patel YA 1985 Ectopic pregnancies: five years hospital experience. *The Practitioner,* 229, March: 269–271

Reynolds M 1984 *Gynaecological nursing.* Blackwell Scientific Publications, London

Ridgeway V & Mathews A 1982 Psychological preparation for Surgery: A comparison of methods. *British Journal of Clinical Psychology,* 21: 271–280

Rogers ME 1970 *An introduction to a theoretical basis of nursing.* F.A. Davis Company, Philadelphia

Roper N 1976 A model for nursing and nursology. *Journal of Advanced Nursing,* 1: 219–227

Roper N, Logan WW & Tierney AJ 1980 *The elements of nursing.* Churchill Livingstone, Edinburgh

Roper N, Logan WW & Tierney AJ 1981 *Learning to use the process of nursing.* Churchill Livingstone, Edinburgh

Roper N, Logan WW & Tierney AJ (Eds) 1983 *Using a model for nursing.* Churchill Livingstone, Edinburgh

Roper N, Logan WW & Tierney AJ 1983 Nursing Process–4–Identifying the Goals. *Nursing Mirror,* 15th June: 22–23

Roy SC 1970 Adaptation: a conceptual framework for nursing. *Nursing Outlook*: 42–45

Speck P 1978 *Loss and grief in medicine.* Ballière Tindall, London

UKCC 1984 *Code of professional conduct for the nurse, midwife and health visitor* (2nd edition) UKCC, London

Webb C 1984 Women's health care in the USA. *Senior Nurse,* 1, 31: 12–13

Webb C 1984 On the eighth day God created the nursing process and nobody rested! *Senior Nurse,* 1, 33: 22–25

Webb C & Wilson Barnett J 1983 Hysterectomy: Dispelling the myths. 2. *Nursing Times* Occasional papers, 79, 31: 44–46

Weinstein L, Morris MB, Dotters D & Christian CD 1983 Ectopic pregnancy–a new surgical epidemic. *Obstetrics and Gynaecology,* 61, 6: 698–701

Westrom L 1975 Effect of acute pelvic inflammatory disease on fertility. *American Journal of Obstetrics and Gynecology,* 121, 5: 707–713

Westrom L, Bengtsson LP, Marsh PA 1981 Incidence, trends and risks of ectopic pregnancy in a population of women. *British Medical Journal,* 282: 15–18

Wilson-Barnett J 1979 *Stress in hospital: patients' psychological reactions to illness and health Care.* Churchill Livingstone, Edinburgh

8

Care plan for a woman having an abdominal hysterectomy, based on Roy's Adaptation model

Christine Webb

This chapter presents a nursing care plan for a patient undergoing abdominal hysterectomy with ovarian conservation and is based on the Roy Adaptation Model (Roy 1980). The discussion begins with an overview of research into recovery from hysterectomy, and goes on to justify the choice of model. A brief explanation of the model is then followed by a critique which leads to modifications in the basic model to enable it to be used as the basis of the care plan. First and second level assessments of the patient are given, together with a care plan for specific teaching and counselling related to hysterectomy. Pre- and post-operative care concerned with patient safety under anaesthetic and physical care are not given, but the use of a standard care plan is suggested to complement the teaching plan. Management and teaching aspects of the use of the model are evaluated and further critical comments are made.

Research into recovery from hysterectomy

Hysterectomy has been a subject of interest to medical writers throughout this century, with gynaecologists' and psychiatrists' contributions to the literature being based on personal views and/or research studies. Whichever kind of report is being read, however, femininity, depression and sexual satisfaction after operation stand out as the main concerns.

Depression is reported to be a fairly common aftermath, its incidence varying from 4 per cent of patients being diagnosed as depressed by a psychiatrist (Melody 1962) to 70 per cent of a general practitioner's patients being given this diagnosis (Richards 1974). Some writers attribute post-hysterectomy depression to oestrogen deficiency (Richards 1974, Wren 1978) but recent research using hormone assays, vaginal cytology to study oestrogen levels indirectly, and measurement of ovarian function by means of radioactive isotopes has shown that oestrogen levels are not changed by hysterectomy alone, without ovarian surgery (Janson & Janson 1977, Coppen *et al.* 1981). Others have put forward a psychosocial explanation for post-hysterectomy depression, describing it as a grief reaction to the loss of an organ which symbolises femininity for women. The suggestion is that a woman's self-concept as a whole and feminine person is damaged when the uterus is removed. Women then no longer perceive themselves as *real* women and the reactions of significant others may reinforce their fears (Green 1973, Raphael 1978). 'Old wives' tales' are one route by which people acquire expectations about the possible results of hysterectomy, and when women waiting to have the operation hear that they may age rapidly, grow facial hair, lose their sexual desire and be an unrewarding sexual partner the tale may turn out to be a self-fulfilling prophecy (Webb & Wilson-Barnett 1983c). At the very least such tales will make women and those close to them anxious about the repercussions of hysterectomy and unsure of what to expect during their recovery.

The medical literature on hysterectomy is open to a number of criticisms, however, some of which have been hinted at already. Different criteria for the diagnosis of depression make comparisons between studies impossible, some reports are speculative and anecdotal rather than research-based, and some research reports include assumptions or values which are not supported by evidence. For example Richards' (1974) conclusion that depression is caused by oestrogen deficiency is not based on measures of oestrogen levels, but rather on his personal observations that prescribing oestrogen tablets for patients was more effective than giving tranquillisers. However, Richards did not conduct a double-blind trial and his own expectations could have influenced both his judgements and the patients' reactions, and the medication could have had a placebo effect.

Recent research with a sound methodological grounding has raised serious doubts about whether hysterectomy does in fact cause depression. Standardised depression measures were used both by Gath (1980) and Coppen *et al.* (1981), and they found *lower* levels of depression after hysterectomy than before. This improvement may result from the relief women feel when they are freed from heavy, irregular bleeding which causes embarrassment, interferes with family, work and social life, and detracts from sexual pleasure.

Webb and Wilson-Barnett (1983a, b, c) looked at depression, self-concept and sexual life during recovery from hysterectomy as part of a nursing study. Research tools included the Beck Depression Inventory (Beck *et al.* 1961), a Mood Adjective Check List to evaluate Anxiety, Fatigue, Hostility and Vigour (Lishman 1972) and a Self-concept Scale (Pearlin & Schooler 1978). Scores on these established instruments confirmed what women told the researchers in interviews carried out one week and four months after hysterectomy. Women felt physically and emotionally much better, were less tired and irritable, had gone back to work, and had

resumed leisure and social activities. Of the 128 women in the study 103 were pre-menopausal at the time of operation, and 94 per cent of these were happy to have no more periods, while 84 per cent were glad that they could no longer become pregnant. Of the 102 sexually active interviewees 90 per cent said their sex life was now as good as or better than previously, and 92 per cent (N = 128) were glad they had had the operation. The small numbers who gave 'negative' replies to these questions were still not completely recovered and gave this as the reason for their answer. They had had complications such as wound, urine or vaginal infections which had delayed recuperation, and so their problems were physical in origin and not psychological as suggested in earlier medical research.

Social support of women recovering from hysterectomy was another variable included in Webb and Wilson-Barnett's study. Social support was defined as a resource for women which, if positive, may aid recovery while negative support will have the opposite effect. Social support resources examined in this research included information given by hospital staff to patients, emotional and physical help given by partners and families, and information in the form of 'old wives' tales'. 'Old wives' tales' giving pessimistic forebodings had been told to 70 per cent of patients (N = 128) but after their own experiences only 11 per cent felt there could be any truth in them. Nevertheless the tales had caused much anxiety and distress until time had proved them false. Women and their partners, families and friends had not talked much about recovery and in approximately half of these cases nobody had made any comment at all about this during the four post-operative months, as far as the women could recall. Partners had taken an average of 1.3 weeks off work after the woman's discharge from hospital, but 23 per cent of partners (N = 103) had given no extra help at all in the home. Information from doctors and nurses was perhaps the greatest area of dissatisfaction expressed by the interviewees, who often made this criticism spontaneously before the researcher posed the relevant question. Twenty per cent (N = 128) were unable to remember being given any advice in preparation for discharge from hospital, and when advice was given it was very brief and focussed only on activities to be avoided. Women would have liked guidance on what they *could* do, how they might *feel* as they progressed, and what symptoms or complications could occur. They felt that warnings about possible problems did not cause anxiety but, on the contrary, were a relief because if a problem arose they would be less afraid and better equipped to deal with it.

In summary, recent studies of recovery from hysterectomy have been well-designed and therefore allow confidence in their findings that women's depression is relieved after hysterectomy and that they do not feel mutilated or less feminine afterwards. Webb and Wilson-Barnett's nursing study provides information for understanding how the process of recovery affects women, what kinds of information they find helpful, and how their coping resources might be augmented through joint counselling of women, their partners and close family members.

Choosing an appropriate model

With this background information about how hysterectomy is experienced by women, the patient chosen for the care plan was considered in order to decide which model of nursing would give the most appropriate guidance in formulating a plan of care. Mrs Mary Smith was 42 years old, had been married for 19 years, and had a son John, aged 17 years, and a daughter Liz, of 15 years of age. The two children were both still at school. Mr Smith was an electrician at a local firm and Mary worked part-time for 20 hours each week as an accounts clerk. Her sister Joan lived with her family 2 miles away from the Smiths, and both their parents were dead. Mary's and Joan's mother had had a hysterectomy when they were teenagers and they remembered her convalescence as a long, drawn-out process punctuated by spells of depression, but felt that their father's death from a heart attack a year earlier could have been an important factor influencing their mother's recovery. Mary had suffered from heavy periods for 18 months. The continual tiredness and unpredictability of her irregular cycles were accompanied by dysmenorrhoea, at which time she passed large clots of blood; these difficulties had led to her ambivalent attitude of both fearing and wanting a hysterectomy. A year prior to her admission she had been told that she had fibroids but had been reluctant to consider surgery until the problem had become virtually unmanageable for her. When seen in the Outpatients Department she had expressed concern to the gynaecologist that she might feel "less of a woman' after hysterectomy because she had heard a lot of stories from colleagues at work and could remember the distress her mother had gone through.

Roy's Adaptation Model (Roy 1980, Rambo 1984) seemed to be the most appropriate choice on which to base Mary's care plan because it considers the biological, psychological and social subsystems which inter-relate to make a human being, and it places a particular emphasis on social roles and the self-concept. This seemed relevant to hysterectomy because research suggested that women fear their self-concept as a feminine person might be damaged when they were no longer able to carry out their reproductive roles. Stories about changes in sexual roles seemed to influence women's expectations, and contacts with family, friends and acquaintances could reinforce these fears. Thus, the focus on self-concept, role function and interdependence in the Roy model were applicable; the underlying pathology of fibroids which leads to physiological disturbances of menstruation and the possibility of complications such as anaemia was included in the physiological mode.

An Activities of Daily Living (ADL) model seemed inappropriate because, although Mary's life had been made miserable by her condition, she was still able to carry out all ADLs without assistance and her operation would only briefly interfere with personal activities. Orem's self-care model appeared less useful too because, except for a few days post-operatively, Mary would be able to be self-caring (Orem 1971).

Therefore, because its concepts fitted so neatly with what research had to say about hysterectomy, Roy's model was selected. Before showing how Mary's nursing assessment was carried out, it is necessary to present an outline of the model and consider whether any modifications are needed in this particular instance.

Elements of Roy's nursing model

The Roy Adaptation Model (Roy 1980, Mastal & Hammond 1980) is based on the assumption that a person is a totality comprised of biological, psychological and social subsystems and that the person is in constant interaction with the changing environment. Multiple stimuli from the environment are encountered by the person, who responds in either adaptive or maladaptive ways. Adaptive responses are those which conserve energy for response to other stimuli, whereas maladaptive responses focus energy in a wasteful and inefficient manner which will lead not to positive adaptation but to coping activity that is inadequate to maintain the integrity of the person in the face of stress.

Roy identifies four modes of acting or adapting, which may also be thought of as four basic areas of need, and these are the *physiological, self-concept, role function and interdependence* modes. In planning nursing care, the person's adaptive level of behaviour in each of the modes is assessed in a primary assessment and then, in a second level assessment, the nurse analyses the stimuli or stressors which are causing the person's need deficit or excess. These stressors or stimuli consist of the immediate or *focal* stimulus causing the problem, *contextual* stimuli which are those present in the environment and which impinge on the present, and *residual* stimuli or beliefs, attitudes and past experiences which are the background influences on the presenting situation. Having identified these stimuli the nurse can then go on to state the patient's or client's present problems, select the goals to be achieved by nursing care, and plan the nursing interven-

tion aimed at bringing about the desired changes or adaptations on the part of the patient/client.

The role of the nurse as conceptualised by Roy is to manipulate the stimuli in order to bring about positive adaptation by the patient. In doing this the nurse supports and promotes patient/client adaptation so that energy is conserved and made available for the healing process rather than being dissipated and used in non-constructive ways.

This brief explanation of the model highlights a number of aspects which need to be questioned and modified before the model can be used as a basis for nursing Mary Smith. One problem has in fact already been dealt with in the presentation because Roy's language has been changed into a gender-neutral form. Roy and the majority of other nursing theorists including King, Orem and Rogers, talk about *man* as the focus of their theories (McFarlane 1980) and this usage is awkward when considering a female patient or client. However, the difficulty is much more profound than simple awkwardness of expression. Words are the building blocks of concepts and therefore the words we use determine the nature of the concepts formed and used to think with. So talking about 'man' is in fact thinking about the men and not women. This plainly is not appropriate and, in the interests of scientific rigour and accuracy, it is important to use gender-neutral language (Moulton 1981, Webb 1983).

The second problem with Roy's model is also related to the use of words and the concepts they indicate, but in this case it is the idea of the nurse manipulating the patient which is ethically questionable. Although Roy (1980) states that the model is patient-centred and the role of the nurse is to support and promote adaptation, a clear emphasis is place on *manipulation* by the nurse and *adaptation* by the patient. Other theorists such as King and Orem emphasise cooperation between nurse and patient and the importance of thinking and acting in terms of the patient's own frame of reference, understanding and self-defined needs. This approach seems appropriate to all nursing situations and particularly to Mary Smith and her forthcoming hysterectomy. In this example it is precisely the frame of reference, beliefs and values of Mary and those close to her which are exacerbating her fears and apprehensions and, if the nurse does not understand these and adapt her care plans accordingly, it is difficult to see how she will help Mary. Thus it is not just the patient who must adapt, but also the nurse and the patient's family and associates, and notions of manipulation seem out of place in this or indeed any humanitarian context.

A further question arises concerning definitions of successful adaptation and who decides what is appropriate adaptation. In research with surgical patients, Cohen and Lazarus (1973) found that patients who tried to exert some control over their own treatment by requesting analgesics progressed less rapidly than those who remained passive, and nurses categorised them as having more psychological problems. This suggests that passivity on the part of the patient would be a positive form of adaptation after surgery. However, most nurses would not want to accept this as desirable and would consider it preferable to change the hospital environment so that patients are encouraged to participate in controlling their own recovery. Surely something is very wrong when patients who are passive in hospital are seen to be making a better adaptation? From the point of view of Mary Smith's family a successful adaptation might be for her to come home from hospital and tire herself out by trying to resume her full housekeeping role immediately, so that they were as little inconvenienced as possible by her operation. Neither Mary nor her nurse would view this as positive adaptation. From a medical point of view, a prescription for tranquillisers might lead to adaptation in the sense of reducing Mary's anxiety, but this would not be positive adaptation in the sense of dealing with the underlying problem. Successful adaptation, then, is a value-laden issue and the question must always be asked, 'For whom is the adaptation positive?'

Roy's choice of words is not accidental but is due to the underlying philosophy of science on which the model is based (Stevens 1979). The model is explained by McFarlane (1980:3) as a scientific theory concerned with 'understanding,

predicting and controlling'. This view of scientific theory, which is often called the 'positivist' view, sees all 'science' as having the same basic characteristics, which are those first established as the procedures of 'hard' sciences such as physics and chemistry. Early social scientists dealing with human phenomena sought to imitate the methods of 'hard' or 'real' science in order to establish the reputation of their disciplines as 'scientific'. Later social scientists considered that different approaches were more appropriate when studying people rather than objects and animals, and that these so-called 'softer' methods were no less scientific but simply were different methods suited to the different subject matter (Melia 1983). It is also argued that 'hard' methods which are concerned with predicting behaviour in order to control it are morally questionable and that this kind of manipulation should not be disguised as neutral, objective science when it actually has these underlying political/moral precepts (Fay 1975, Spencer 1983). This short discussion of the philosophical basis of science cannot begin to do justice to the complexity of the issues involved but it does raise questions about Roy's philosophy of nursing which merit deeper consideration when deciding whether the model is an acceptable foundation for planning nursing care.

Certain modifications are therefore needed in Roy's model before it can be used as the basis for Mary Smith's care. The need for mutuality and reciprocity between nurse and patient must be accepted, and the two should agree together on a definition of problems and which stimuli they will manipulate together in order to try to reach agreed goals. Otherwise the nurse may set unattainable goals and might inadvertently alienate her patient rather than helping her to cope with the stressful situation she is facing. In this situation it is not only the patient who is affected by the stressor, and so her family needs to be included in the adaptation process. Indeed in this example the patient's family is part of the stressful situation and to ignore them would detract from the possibility of successfully helping Mary to adapt.

On the basis of this modified version of Roy's

adaptation model, first and second level assessments of Mary Smith can be made, and these are given in Figure 8.1. A minimum of discussion should be needed to explain these assessments because all the necessary information ought to be contained in the assessment itself and in the resulting care plan, which is given in Figure 8.2. When nurses use the care plan they should be able to proceed on its basis alone as often the person who carried out the assessment and drew up the care plan will not be available for consultation. Therefore the documentation should be complete and should be able to stand alone without the need for additional material. Mary Smith's principal problems are identified as lack of accurate and realistic information about the details of her operation, its likely effects and non-effects, and how she and her family will cope in the convalescent phase. Therefore the care plan presented focuses on the information-giving and counselling aspects of her care, and the details of her pre- and post-operative care are not given in the interests of saving space. Nurses justifiably express concern that care planning can become a time-consuming process which takes them away from the essential aspects of patient care. Such reservations are especially valid on wards such as gynaecology, where patients' stays can be quite short and many patients have similar core needs and problems. Standard care plans for pre- and post-operative care concerned with aspects of patient safety under anaesthetic seem justified in this situation, with patients' particular needs being catered for by a supplementary care plan of the type under discussion in this chapter.

Teaching and management implications

The teaching style used to implement the care plan is vital to its success, and both the information-giving and counselling aspects need to be considered. Information-giving must meet the patient's own level of understanding and employ language which is meaningful to her, and this involves individual judgement as the nurse gets to know the patient. Through talking to her conversationally and while taking her nursing history the nurse will form impressions of how much her patient already understands, where knowledge gaps exist, and where misinformation needs correction. She will also hear the kind of language the patient uses and will be able to decide whether to use the same terminology, for example whether to say 'womb' for 'uterus' or 'neck of womb' instead of 'cervix', and will be able to judge which technical terms require an explanation (Lion 1982). It is not always useful simply to use lay terminology without explaining technical terms, because patients may feel more comfortable talking to staff, in particular doctors, in medical terms and may appreciate learning these in order to employ them correctly in future.

Research has shown that people remember medical information best when the importance of items is stressed, when information is repeated and reinforced, and when it is backed up by a written record (Ley 1977). Psychological theory relating to memory, forgetting and timespan of concentration suggests that short informational inputs followed by breaks or rests, and punctuated by rehearsals of what has been learned increase the amount remembered (Rogers 1971). Information-giving to patients, therefore, must be carefully programmed so that overloading is avoided and patients are not given so much information at one time that they cannot retain it. Advice cannot be followed if it is forgotten and so the teaching suggested in the care plan should be spread over Mary's stay in hospital, integrated with other care, and presented at the relevant stage. For example, information about pre- and post-operative care and teaching of exercises must be done before operation, but discharge planning discussions might be delayed until the patient is feeling better after her operation.

Teaching needs to be complemented by a counselling approach in which nurse and patient develop a two-way relationship of trust and understanding so that the patient feels able to ask any questions, no matter how 'silly' or simple they may seem. Through an informal approach, the use of eye-contact and 'constructive listening' techniques the patient comes to feel comfortable in sharing her emotions with the nurse, and this provides not only a way of discharging tension but also gives the nurse additional opportunities to pick up cues about how the patient feels, and her needs for information and support (Bridge & MacLeod Clark 1981, Webb & Wilson-Barnett 1983c).

Audio-visual aids to accompany teaching can stimulate attention by adding variety to the presentation and helping the patient to understand ideas that are difficult to express in words. Posters showing the anatomy of the pelvis or a smaller diagram from a book are essential, but in addition nurses can involve medical staff, physiotherapists, dietitians and others in writing information leaflets for patients to keep for reference at home. A number of information leaflets and booklets for hysterectomy patients have already been produced by nurses and others and these might be adopted, possibly with modifications to suit the particular situation (Steele & Goodwin 1975, Carter 1981, Savage 1982, Haslett & Jennings). A tape-recording might be made of a nurse talking to a former patient who has had a full recovery; an even more ambitious idea would be to make a tape-slide programme for patients to use singly or in groups, accompanied by discussion with a nurse.

Ward management issues need to be considered because teaching must be seen as a fundamental part of nursing care for which time is allowed. A systematic strategy for carrying out teaching also needs to be developed. In Mary Smith's case primary nursing seems to offer a way of personalising teaching and helping nurses and the patient to develop the kind of confiding relationship which is essential to a counselling-style approach. Primary nursing allows continuity so that the plan is effectively carried out (Pearson 1983). A primary nurse would be assigned to Mary on admission and would conduct her nursing assessment and devise the care plan. Associate nurses would be allocated for back-up when the primary nurse is not on duty. They would follow the care plan and discuss their observations, progress and any suggested

modifications with the primary nurse, who would retain responsibility for adapting the plan and ensuring that it is carried out.

Evaluating the approach: a critique of the model in use

The earlier critical evaluation of Roy's model can be further developed after devising and testing the care plan. Mastal and Hammond (1980) state that the scientific basis of the model is vague, and this criticism was borne out when attempting to carry out the first level assessment. Social psychological work on the self-concept emphasises its essentially social aspects and the fact that the self-concept develops and is modified via verbal and non-verbal messages from significant others (Garrity *et al.* 1977). This makes Roy's separation of self-concept, role function and interdependence into three different modes difficult to justify theoretically and to apply in practice. Dilemmas therefore arose over Mary's guilt about temporarily abandoning her family while she was in hospital: should this be placed under the heading self-concept, role function or interdependence? Similar questions arose in relation to her anxiety about being too demanding of nurses: was this a self-concept or interdependence item? Did her fears about post-operative sex life relate to all three modes or not? In practice, decisions tended to be made arbitrarily and other variations could be equally justifiable.

Lack of criteria for operationalising concepts was referred to earlier, and personal values about 'adaptation' are inevitably reflected in the care plan in the absence of precise guidelines. An attempt was made to 'manipulate' Mary's family into helping her, based on the judgement that her needs should be given greater priority than theirs at this time. Other possible ways of manipulating the situation are imaginable, such as trying to arrange a stay in a convalescent home or a home help to provide Mary with the chance to give priority to her personal recovery in the early weeks. The model gives no help in making these decisions because 'adaptation' is left undefined and is probably undefinable except on the basis of individual value preferences influenced by cultural norms and values.

In conclusion, the use of Roy's adaptation model to plan care for this patient undergoing hysterectomy had the advantage of providing some structure for assessment and planning, and this helped to ensure that all her needs were considered. Theoretical criticisms of model were validated in practice, and without certain modifi-

cations the patient's care would have been incomplete and ineffective because her husband and family would have been omitted from the intervention.

Further development of the model is required to allow its operationalisation but, even if this were to be done, fundamental ethical questions relating to notions of control, manipulation and the role of the nurse mean that its acceptance as a basis for nursing care is problematic.

Fig. 8.1 First and second level assessment of patient based on Roy's Adaptation Model (Roy 1980)

	First Level Assessment	Second Level Assessment		
		Focal stimuli	Contextual stimuli	Residual stimuli
Physiological Mode				
Exercise and rest	Has been getting very tired and irritable recently because of heavy and irregular bleeding. Goes to work by bus now, but used to cycle. Sleeps well: 11 pm to 7 am.	Fibroids, causing heavy bleeding	Aged 42, housewife and part-time clerk.	
Nutrition	Has been 'comfort eating', and put on 16 pounds in weight in past 6 months.	Heavy, irregular bleeding and associated anxiety		Cultural definitions of healthy nutrition
Elimination	Urinary system: no problems. Bowels: tendency to constipation. Has All Bran for breakfast to control this.	Lack of fibre in diet		
Fluid and electrolytes	Normal hydration.			
Oxygen	Respirations: 14 per minute, no cough. Colour: normal.			
Circulation	Pulse: 66 per minute, regular, good volume. No oedema.			
Regulation				
a Temperature	36.8° C orally.			
b Senses	Vision, hearing, taste, touch, smell all normal.			
c Endocrine system	Has pre-menstrual syndrome; bloated feeling in abdomen and sore breasts before menstruation, worse in past year. Hopes hysterectomy will relieve this.	Possible hormone imbalance associated with heavy bleeding		
Self-concept mode				
Physical	Wonders if she will feel any different when there is 'an empty space inside' after operation. Afraid of anaesthetic and of not waking up afterwards.	Impending hysterectomy. No previous anaesthetic	Has been told 'old wives' tales' by women at work	Remembers mother's difficult recovery from hysterectomy.

Personal	Worried that hysterectomy will alter her 'feelings of being a woman' but relieved not to be fertile afterwards.	Impending hysterectomy	As above	As above. Cultural values of feminity.
Inter-personal self	Anxious about asking nurses for help in case she is being a 'nuisance'.	As above	As above	General beliefs that nurses are always busy, patients should not be demanding.
Role function mode				
Role failure	Afraid that she will not be able to give her husband sexual satisfaction after operation.	As above	As above	
	Afraid that it may take a long time to get back to usual standards of housekeeping and return to work.	As above	As above	Cultural expectations about women's work.
Role conflict	Feels guilty about leaving husband and family to cope at home, but realises that she needs to sort out her own health problems. No religious conflicts.	As above	As above	As above
Interdependence mode				
	Worried about husband's reaction to the possible sexual effects of operation. Feels that husband and family do not realise what a big operation hysterectomy is and will expect her to get straight back to normal when she goes home.	As above	Family do not usually 'help' much in the home and she is proud to manage herself.	As above
	Glad to have her sister's understanding and sympathy. The sisters are very close to each other.	As above	Sister has offered to help and has talked to Mary about the operation.	Memories of mother's hysterectomy

Fig. 8.2 Individual care plan for Mary Smith

Problem (P) Potential (A) Actual	Goal	Intervention	Evaluation Criteria
(A) Anxiety about possible effect of hysterectomy, due to inadequate information	Reduce anxiety to levels which do not disturb Mary by giving information to promote understanding	Explain, with the help of a simple diagram, the operation and its effects and non-effects: parts removed and remaining continued hormone production loss of menstruation and fertility vagina and outer organs remain intact sexual activity will not change and may improve as general health is better cervical smears no longer necessary	Mary: is able to repeat explanation to partner demonstrates understanding in conversations with staff and patients says she is less anxious about having operation
(A) Fear of actual operation process, and having anaesthetic (NB some fear is realistic and expected)	Reduce anxiety to levels which do not disturb Mary by giving information to promote understanding and control	Explain pre- and post-operative procedures Encourage patient to ask for help from staff, e.g. analgesia, anti-emetics, assistance to bathroom	Mary: answers check questions correctly asks questions asks for medication when needed practises exercises says she is less anxious about having operation
(A) Anxiety about progress after discharge due to memories of mother's hysterectomy and hearing 'old wives' tales'	Mary will feel confident in controlling her own recovery	Stress that progress is individual and comparison with others is not useful. Suggest using own feelings and tiredness levels to guide progress. Suggest for the first 2 weeks at home: getting up late and going to bed early getting dressed during the day resting with feet up in the afternoon going for short, gradually increasing walks avoiding all but the lightest housework. Mention 'old wives' tales' and refute their accuracy	Mary: makes plans for convalescence and discusses them with nurse and other patients talks to family about her needs for help discusses the tales she has heard and questions their truth

Problem	Goal	Nursing action	Outcome
		Warn about possible experiences and advise on appropriate action: tiredness, pain, feeling 'low'. Explain measure to avoid: constipation – high fibre diet weight gain – high fibre, low fat, low calorie diet, exercise depression – talk to family and friends about feelings, avoid being alone all the time. Advise consulting GP in the case of: vaginal discharge which is increased in amount, has unpleasant smell, is blood-stained or frankly red burning or difficulty on passing urine leaking operation wound	
(A) Low expectation of help with housekeeping from husband and family	Mary will ask for and receive guarantees of appropriate help	Talk to husband and children at visiting time, repeating advice given to Mary and suggesting they talk about how the home will be run in the early post-discharge weeks	Mary and family: discuss patient's needs and share out responsibilities for household jobs ask for information and advice from nurse
(P) Constipation after operation	Regular, pain-free soft bowel action from 3rd day post-operatively	Check Mary's understanding of fibre-rich foods Give dietary advice leaflet Ask doctor to prescribe aperient for post-operative use if needed Check dietary intake Assist to lavatory when desired Give medication or suppositories if needed	Mary: chooses high fibre diet from menu has regular, pain-free, soft bowel action from 3rd day post-operatively
(P) Disappointment if pre-menstrual tension is not relieved after hysterectomy	Mary will understand that hormone production will go on and that PMT may still occur	Explain that ovaries will be retained to avoid an early menopause Warn that PMT may still occur but may be less severe	Mary: answers check questions correctly asks questions

References

Beck AT, Ward CH, Mendelson M, Mock J & Erbaugh J 1961 An inventory for measuring depression. *Archives of General Psychiatry*, **4**: 561–571

Bridge W & MacLeod Clark J 1981 *Communication in nursing care*. HM and M, London

Carter S 1981 Ready for home? *Nursing Times*, May 7: 826–829

Cohen F & Lazarus 1973 Active coping processes, coping dispositions and recovery from surgery. *Psychosomatic Medicine*, **35**: 375–389

Coppen A, Bishop M, Beard RJ, Barnard GJR & Collins WP 1981 Hysterectomy, hormones and behaviour. *Lancet*, Jan 17: 126–128

Fay B 1975 *Social theory and political practice*. Allen and Unwin, London

Garrity, TF, Somes GW & Marx MB 1977 Personality factors in resistance to illness after recent life changes. *Journal of Psychosomatic Research*, **21**: 23–32

Gath D 1980 Psychiatric aspects of hysterectomy. In: Rubins L, Clayton P, Wing J (Eds) *The social consequences of psychiatric illness*. Brunner-Mazel Inc., New York

Green RL 1973 The emotional aspects of hysterectomy. *Southern Medical Journal*, **66**: 442–444

Haslett S & Jennings M (No date) *Hysterectomy and vaginal repair*. Johnson and Johnson Ltd., Slough

Janson PE & Janson I 1977 The acute effect of hysterectomy on ovarian bloodflow. *American Journal of Obstetrics and Gynecology*, **127**:349–352

Ley P 1977 Psychologic studies in doctor–patient communication. In: Rachman S (Ed) *Contributions to medical psychology*, 1. Pergamon Press, Oxford

Lion EM (Ed) 1982 *Human sexuality in nursing process*. J Wiley, New York

Lishman WA 1972 Selective factors in memory. Part 2. Affective disorders. *Psychological Medicine*, **2**: 248–253

Mastal MF & Hammond H 1980 Analysis and expansion of the Roy adaption model: a contribution to holistic nursing. *Advances in Nursing Science*, **20**, 4: 71–81

McFarlane EA 1980 Nursing theory: the comparison of four theoretical proposals. *Journal of Advanced Nursing*, **5**: 3–19

Melia K 1983 Students' views of nursing. *Nursing Times*, May 18: 24–25

Melody GR 1962 Depressive reactions following hysterectomy. *American Journal of Obstetrics and Gynecology*, **83**: 410–413

Moulton J 1981 The myth of the neutral 'man'. In: Vetterling-Braggin M (Ed) *Sexist language: a modern philosophical analysis*. Littlefield, Adams and Co., Totowa, NJ

Orem D 1971 *Nursing: concepts of practice*. McGraw-Hill, New York

Pearlin IL & Schooler C 1978 The structure of coping. *Journal of Health and Social Behavior*, March 19: 2–21

Pearson A 1983 *The clinical nursing unit*. Heinemann, London

Rambo B 1984 *Adaptation nursing. Assessment and intervention*. Saunders, Philadelphia

Raphael B 1978 Psychiatric aspects of hysterectomy. In: Howell JG (Ed) *Modern perspectives in the psychiatric aspects of surgery*. Macmillan, London

Richards DH 1974 A post-hysterectomy syndrome. *Lancet*, October 26: 983–985

Rogers J 1971 *Adults learning*. Open University, Milton Keynes

Roy C 1980 The Roy adaptation model. In: Riehl J and Roy C (Eds) *Conceptual models for nursing practice*. Appleton-Century-Crofts, New York

Savage W 1982 *Hysterectomy*. Hamlyn Paperbacks, London

Spencer J 1983 Research with a human touch. *Nursing Times*, May 18: 24–27

Steele S J & Goodwin MF 1975 A pamphlet to answer the patient's questions before hysterectomy. *Lancet*, September 13: 492–493

Stevens B J 1979 *Nursing theory*. Little, Brown and Company, Boston

Webb C 1983 Words fail me. *Nursing Times*, July 6: 65–66

Webb C & Wilson-Barnett J 1983a Self-concept, social support and hysterectomy. *International Journal of Nursing Studies*, **20**, 2: 97–107

Webb C & Wilson-Barnett J 1983b Coping with hysterectomy. *Journal of Advanced Nursing*, **8**, 3: 311–319

Webb C & Wilson-Barnett J 1983c Hysterectomy: dispelling the myths. Part 1 and Part 2. *Nursing Times* **79**, 30; Occasional Paper: 52–54 and **79**, 31: Occasional Paper: 44–46

Wren B 1978 Counselling the hysterectomy patient. *Medical Journal of Australia*, **1**: 87–189

9

Care plan for a woman having a vaginal hysterectomy, based on Roper's Activities of Living model

Ann Webb

This chapter presents a nursing care plan for an older woman undergoing vaginal hysterectomy for prolapse. The care plan is based on Roper's model as laid out in *The Elements of Nursing* (Roper, Logan & Tierney 1980), and is written from a health visiting perspective. Relevant research on hysterectomy and repair for prolapse, the use of the vaginal route as opposed to the abdominal route, and subsequent recovery are discussed. An outline of the model follows, together with a critical evaluation of the use of the model and its value as a teaching tool.

Research into vaginal hysterectomy

For many years medical researchers have lamented the fact that there is no standard means of assessing the patient's recovery after hysterectomy (Jones & Doyle 1943, Dicker *et al.* 1982). It is only in recent years that nursing research has begun to look at this area and has met similar difficulties. Most researchers use their own means of assessing and monitoring recovery, and comparisons of results are not easy (Gould 1985). Precise difficulties in comparison and methodological defects are covered comprehensively in a study of 'Self-concept, social support and hysterectomy' by Webb and Wilson-Barnett (1983). Medical research into vaginal hysterectomy or repair provides an interesting debate. It also raises issues, some controversial, that may have repercussions on patients' recovery.

The technique of vaginal hysterectomy was first perfected and used by the French and then the Germans between 1800–1900, but it was not popular practice in Britain until around 1950. The 17th British Obstetric and Gynaecological Conference held in Glasgow in 1965 discussed vaginal surgery, and a mass of medical opinion and research was presented to the conference about the vaginal route for hysterectomy in preference to the abdominal route.

A study by Gudex (1965) compared 200 vaginal and 200 abdominal hysterectomies. He concluded that improved vaginal technique had resulted in a decreased post-operative morbidity and that urinary complications were related to catheterisation and not to the mode of operation.

Stirling (1965) summarised his surgical experience of vaginal hysterectomy as part of a repair procedure as being satisfactory. Others agreed that it was tolerated well by the patient, involved few of the risks attached to, and took less time than, the abdominal route (Navratil 1965). Improved techniques meant that shock was less frequent and hospital stay was reduced (Steptoe 1965). Its use decreased the incidence of serious complications and made post-operative recovery more comparable to that after a minor surgical procedure as opposed to the major surgery of the abdominal route (Weaver 1965).

The ethics of removing a healthy womb at the time of repairing a prolapse were also widely debated. Those in favour of vaginal hysterectomy and repair saw the repair as producing the complications (Stirling 1965, Weaver 1965).

Weaver was outspoken in his view that a repair without hysterectomy was an 'incomplete operation' and that Manchester Repair would soon be a thing of the past. There were dissenting views, however, and Morris (1965) stated that his patients preferred a repair and were very reluctant to part with their healthy wombs. Morris was experienced in the Manchester Repair technique and stated that vaginal hysterectomy was unnecessary for a prolapse with a healthy womb. Stirling (1965) also disagreed with prophylactic removal of healthy wombs except in older women. Several speakers stressed that success and low morbidity depended on the expertise of the surgeon (Navratil 1965, Steptoe 1965, Stirling 1965).

Few studies were available at that time on long-term morbidity and, due to the difficulties of confusing research and opinions, only general conclusions emerged. Thus for women younger than 40 years who wished to have more children, to keep their menstrual function, or who had healthy wombs, repair would be performed. Those women aged 40 and over who needed repair for prolapse would undergo vaginal hysterectomy at the same time, to avoid the possibility of further surgery at a later date for menstrual problems or a diseased uterus.

Many at the conference felt that vaginal hysterectomy allowed a better repair but that, if removal of the womb at a repair operation caused increased occurrence of death or post-operative morbidity, it could not be justified (Hawksworth 1965, Howkins 1965, Stirling 1965, Weaver 1965).

More recent research has reiterated the problems expressed at this conference and also the conclusion that prolapse, especially in older women, is best dealt with by vaginal hysterectomy. Its advantages include a better repair, less post-operative distress, and earlier ambulation and discharge from hospital (Feroze 1977, Dicker *et al.* 1982, Stanton *et al.* 1982). A study by Porges (1980) compared vaginal hysterectomy with vaginal hysterectomy and repair, and the average age of women in the sample was 56 years. Not only was there less bleeding after the combined operation, but long-term follow-up showed no later prolapse of the vaginal vault. Ellenborgen *et al.* (1981) also stressed the value of this combined procedure in older women (over 65 years of age). An expectation of post-operative complications in women of this age was realised, but did not result in extended hospital stays. Roos (1984) found the morbidity rate following both abdominal and vaginal hysterectomy higher than that of cholecystectomy patients, and of women in the general population, and therefore urged careful consideration of the risks and advantages of hysterectomy in elective surgery. Low mortality and morbidity is still seen as dependent on the surgeon's expertise in vaginal surgery (Dennerstein *et al.* 1977, Feroze 1977, Shapiro *et al.* 1982).

Research into recovery from hysterectomy

Conflicting research evidence exists about depression after hysterectomy, mainly due, until recently, to the lack of standard definitions and measuring techniques. Few references take into account the mode of surgery (vaginal or abdominal route) or age. Those that do, reveal that depression is not related to mode of surgery, and that age shows a positive influence, the incidence of depression being lower in older post-menopausal women (Barker 1968, DH Richards 1973).

Studies also show that women need information and explanations to help them prepare for surgery and to make the adjustments necessary for recovery (Boore 1978, Raphael 1978). Yet, few have considered what women prefer, what preparation best equips them for this operation, or their quality of life after discharge from hospital. Keith (1980), writing about a support group for post-hysterectomy patients, described the philosophy of the hospital where the group was based. This was based on the belief that illness or admission to hospital is a threat to the patient's autonomy, and that staff have a responsibility to give information and education to the patient to enable adjustment. Preparation for discharge after hysterectomy at this hospital involves self-care, support and individual coun-selling. Steele and Goodwin (1975) emphasise that information needs to be patient-orientated and not simply the doctor's views. Where women have been involved in making an informed decision about hysterectomy, recovery is re-ported as uneventful and women express satis-faction with the surgery (BC Richards 1978). 'Informed decision-making' in this example in-volved explaining the differences between life-saving hysterectomy, elective hysterectomy and prophylactic hysterectomy. Full discussion of *all* possible risks, advantages and possible alter-natives to hysterectomy also took place. The ma-jority in the sample were classed as 'elective hysterectomies', but the survey was carried out by the patients' own gynaecologist and the classification may therefore be biased.

Recent nursing research has explored some of the issues in this area of hysterectomy. Carter (1981) found that patients required information about hysterectomy that nurse learners were unable to give. Haslett and Jennings (1984) also found a need to provide written information for in-patients before surgery, as part of a counsel-ling service. They devised a booklet based on a study involving several questionnaires to in-patients about the information they would like. Preparation in out-patient clinics, with infor-mation on surgery and discussions of expec-tations and the recovery period, have been found to be successful in reducing post-operative an-xiety (Powell 1982). Pre-operative information about surgery and the recovery period are im-portant for the woman's ability to cope with the trauma of surgery (Kuczynski 1982), and talking through feelings about hysterectomy produces beneficial effects (Webb 1983). Lack of prepar-ation for discharge home is also a problem for patients, who require specific information on gradual resumption of activities (Gould 1985).

Nurses can play a major role in counselling and assessing the individual needs of patients (Wilson-Barnett 1981) and nurses realise this, but lack the training for what is seen to be a post-registration speciality (Webb 1985). Continued support can be provided by community staff through health education and preventive care.

Patient participation in planning their own re-covery is important and aids recovery through reduction of anxiety (Wilson-Barnett 1981; Kuczynski 1982).

Limited data is available about patients' ex-periences at home. Most research has been hospital-based, but several researchers have noted a substantial number of residual physical symptoms several months after surgery (Kuczynski 1982, Gould 1985). High levels of infection after discharge home and complaints of tiredness several months later were reported (Webb 1983). Whether this morbidity can have psychiatric sequelae is a question which needs further research.

Information given in response to women's questions, counselling in conjunction with prac-tical advice, and support from friends and relatives have all been found to affect women's recovery and levels of anxiety (Webb & Wilson-Barnett 1983, Kuczynski 1982). A paper on hysterectomy counselling has described the in-volvement of the health visitor in a self-help support group, and suggests that low self-image and poor self-esteem seem to restrict the use of available information sources and avenues of support before surgery (A Webb 1985). This may well reflect women's acceptance of a patriarchal society's questioning of their right to be self-determining.

C Webb (1985) discusses this suggestion as well as women's sense of isolation and need for information when facing hysterectomy. Control-ling and participating in decisions about what is to happen to one's body are an important part of coping, and provision of information, support and counselling to facilitate this is an area that fits well into the role of the health visitor (A Webb 1985).

In summary, vaginal hysterectomy and repair is the operation of choice for older women with prolapse. There is less depression in older women, but there may be an appreciable physical morbidity post-operatively in comparison with other surgery such as cholecystectomy. Women require more information than is often given to prepare them for surgery and recovery, but where information, support and specific advice are given, then this affects recovery favourably. Involvement in her own care planning is helpful to the woman's coping abilities. Counselling that allows for exchange of information, expression of anxieties and expectations, and involvement of the patient in her own health choices is not only a health visiting priority but an aid to recovery.

The role of the health visitor

The Council for the Education and Training of Health Visitors (CETHV) outlines the basic functions of the health visitor as the prevention of mental, physical, emotional ill health and its consequences, early detection of ill-health and surveillance of high risk groups, recognition and identification of the need and use of appropriate resources, health teaching, the provision of care and support during periods of stress, advice and guidance in illness as well as in the care and management of children. Crow (1981), however, questions the overlap in these criteria and whether they actually reflect what happens in practice.

Health visiting priorities as defined by local health district policy are often heavily weighted in favour of mothers with young babies. However, part of the responsibility and ethos of health visiting is constantly to assess health needs and services in the community, and to heighten individual and social awareness of those needs. The health visitor seeks to facilitate informed health choices and to encourage individuals to be self-determining.

The difficulties in assessing and evaluating health visiting and of the health visitor's reluctance both to use the nursing process and to visit older women are discussed by Luker (1983), yet this group was seen by health visitors in her study as a high risk group. The study shows that older women are very independent, seeing health visitor care as more suitable in times of illness, and Luker suggests that dislike of this type of visiting by the health visitor is rooted in the lack of visiting structure. When visiting mothers and young children the emphasis is on expected milestones of normal development, but this

approach is not suitable for older women for whom gradual deterioration in health is the expectation. There may be an element of insecurity for health visitors working with older women as opposed to advising a mother about her child. When visiting mothers, the advice given is about a third party; when visiting older women, the advice given is to the woman directly. Thus, instant feed-back is received in response, and the health visitor is more likely to be openly challenged about what her role really is. Using a modified form of the nursing process can clarify this both for the health visitor and her client (Clark 1982).

Choosing an appropriate model

In considering which model to use as a basis for care planning there are several factors to take into account. The first of these is the patient herself. The client to be discussed in this chapter is Rose Normandy, a 74 year old single woman who lives alone. She is active and alert, and has in the past been the carer in her extended family. Miss Normandy recently cared for her niece after she had undergone an abdominal hysterectomy. Her family of one brother and sister, their spouses and children all live at great distances from her and each other. Her busy social life includes involvement in local voluntary groups and clubs, and Miss Normandy shops and cooks each Saturday and Sunday for two separate friends, both in their nineties. She experienced no health problems prior to the development of urinary symptoms of urgency and dribbling, which began five years ago. A prolapse was diagnosed and Miss Normandy was told that she was too old for surgery.

After an increase of discomfort and symptoms a ring pessary was fitted two years ago, but it was never checked or removed for cleaning and Miss Normandy received no instructions about this. Intermittent urinary and vaginal infections followed, until six months ago she experienced vaginal bleeding and pain. Miss Normandy went to the Accident and Emergency Department and was admitted to hospital. The ring was removed under a general anaesthetic and Miss Normandy was advised that, when the ulcerations and infection had cleared up, she would be re-admitted for a vaginal hysterectomy.

Miss Normandy had been dismayed at the lack of information given to her niece about her recent hysterectomy, and was concerned about what was involved in a vaginal hysterectomy. She was a reserved, private person who felt that she could not discuss these problems with her distant family or dependent friends, but she eventually expressed her anxiety to a health visitor after a talk about women's health at one of her clubs.

Miss Normandy does not fit into the usual 'researched' group for hysterectomy. She is post-menopausal, with no intimate relationships, and is above the age at which the usual myths would be frightening, including tales that hysterectomy ages you rapidly, gives rise to loss of sexual drive, and makes you masculine (Webb & Wilson-Barnett 1983). It is a normal expectation that Miss Normandy will undergo the gradual de-teriorations in health common with increasing age. Despite initiating the contact, it is probable that Miss Normandy does not fully understand the services of the health visitor (Luker 1983). Her self-expressed needs are for information, and help to arrange suitable care for her de-pendent friends, but these may or may not be the sum total of her anxieties.

The second consideration in choosing a nurs-ing model is the nature of the health visitor's role generally, and in relation to Miss Normandy in particular. This role is more likely to be chal-lenged by an older woman, who will relinquish the service when the perceived crisis is passed. Validation of her role, to herself and to Miss Normandy, may be difficult for the health visitor (Luker 1983). There is also a need to monitor changes in body systems due to age, and the emergence of possible post-operative morbidity after discharge home. Assessment of each, dif-ferentiation between the two, and initiation of appropriate action and use of resources will be important. The work environment is the patient's home and the choice to involve and use

the health visitor is always the patient's. The health visitor seeks to motivate the patient to take control of her own health and to provide infor-mation and encouragement to enable her to assess and plan for her present and future well-being. This involves appropriate use of available services and staff, including the health visitor. Health visitor involvement is long-term unless terminated by the patient as there is no discharge system, and in practice contact often spans several years, with a time lag of varying length between each visit.

In working through the problem of adapting the nursing process for health visiting, Clark (1982) points out that all clients have needs but not all have problems. Older people may have potential problems. Her use of SOAPIER (Subjective, Objective, Assessment, Plan, Intervention, Evaluation, Re-assessment) ad-apted from SOAP (Weed 1969) is based on a developmental framework (Sheridan 1973) which is not applicable to Miss Normandy, an older woman.

A systems model appears to meet most of the requirements of a model in this instance. It allows structured monitoring of Miss Normandy over a period of time and therefore detection of failing abilities or delayed onset of low-grade complications. It also gives a structure to the visit that reveals the wide area of interest that the health visitor has in the individual.

A preliminary look at Johnson's model, with nursing intervention set out in aggressive ter-minology, suggests that it is more suitable for a hospital environment. It is therefore rejected as inappropriate for use in a community setting without major adaptation.

The Roy Adaptation Model looks more prom-ising, in that Miss Normandy may view the validity of her own life through her usefulness to others. If this is so, then her self-image may well be damaged by the enforced relinquishing of her social functions due to undergoing surgery. The model appears to be easily adaptable for use in the community. However, the very strong em-phasis on role-function and self-concept and its complex terminology make it unsuitable as the first choice for use with Miss Normandy.

An Activities of Living (AL) model seems most relevant. It takes in many aspects of health visitor assessment and, with adjustment, fits into a community setting. It gives a structure for working with this age group and a base for discussion and exchange of information between Miss Normandy and the health visitor. Interestingly, the ALs also encompass most of the health problems listed by Luker (1983) as valid check-points around which a health visitor could plan her visit. Through its use, Miss Normandy can be given a clearer idea of the health visiting focus and how many different systems can be affected by surgery. The terminology is straightforward for Miss Normandy to understand and relate to, and the model provides the necessary opportunities to prepare and plan for major surgery and the recovery period.

Elements of Roper's nursing model

Roper laid the foundation of the Activities of Living (AL) model by drawing from the physiological, psychological and nursing sciences to put forward a model of nursing in 1976. Moving away from the disease/medical approach, Roper looked at the process of living, and for ways to assess and understand human beings based on observable behaviour. Certain everyday activities were seen as behavioural manifestations of human needs. Roper, Logan and Tierney's model (1980) is a refined version of this original model and the individual is viewed as a unique being through 12 activities, namely Maintaining a Safe Environment, Communicating, Breathing, Eating and Drinking, Eliminating, Personal Cleansing and Dressing, Controlling Body Temperature, Mobilising, Working and Playing, Expressing Sexuality, Sleeping, and Dying. These activities are further defined as being in one of the categories of preventing, comforting or seeking. Some activities are concerned with the essentials of living, such as breathing, and have a biological base. Some are

non-essential and are concerned with the quality of life, such as cleanliness, and have a social/cultural base. Despite being expressed as part of a list, each activity is complex and is inter-related with others. This can lead to difficulties of classification and possibly to some assessments being incomplete or duplicated. Nevertheless, the advantage of this 'list' for Miss Normandy lies in the structure provided to assess relevant areas of her life and health.

The performance of these twelve activities is influenced by other dimensions of living (Roper, Logan and Tierney 1980). The individual's physical, psychological, emotional and social environments change during each person's life from birth to death, and at various ages people can be totally dependent, partially dependent, or totally independent of help with ALs. Disability or disturbed physiology may present at birth or be acquired, and can result in physical and/or mental dysfunction. Physical changes may be linked with deterioration due to age or disease, while accidents and infections will also bring about changes – some permanent, some temporary. All affect not only the individual's ability to cope with her ALs but also how, when and if the ALs are performed. These make Roper's model of particular relevance to Miss Normandy, who will be facing the changes related to increasing age. The effect of any post-operative morbidity will also influence her moods and perhaps her mental and physical ability to cope with ALs.

In summary, the performance of ALs is influenced by age, by the physical, emotional, psychological environments, levels of dependence, past experiences, cultural and social circumstances, and the individuality of each person. The model's objective is for individuals to reach their full potential in each AL, as permitted by these influencing factors. The ALs are the framework for the nursing process of Assessment, Planning, Nursing Intervention and Evaluation, and documentation is an important part of the process. The aim of nursing intervention is to help the individual achieve the objective stated above, namely maximum independence and well-being.

Information about each AL is required to

assess the patient's situation before planning nursing care. This helps establish previous routines, what the patient can do unaided, what actual problems exist, or what potential problems may develop, and the patient's previous coping systems. From this baseline a list of priorities can be made, with observable and measurable results in terms of patient behaviour.

Planning of appropriate nurse intervention involves setting goals with the patient, and the assessment of available resources. Goals should be described in terms of patient behaviour. Resources include utilisation of the patient's own coping processes, as well as use of voluntary and statutory support services in the community.

Nursing intervention provides help with actual problems with as little disruption as possible to the patient's usual habits, and encourages healthy living in order to avoid potential problems. This help ranges from providing information or equipment to performing a task of living for the patient.

Evaluation involves consideration of the goals set in the planning stage. It is dependent on the specification of observable or measurable behaviour and needs to be set in a time schedule.

This overview of the model leads to several implications for the health visitor and patient which need to be looked at more closely. Some terminology seems more suited to the hospital environment, and the word 'Patient' sits uneasily in the health visitor setting where the emphasis is on prevention of ill-health and the promotion of active good health. The dictionary definition of patient is 'a person under medical or surgical treatment: a physician's client'. In fact the majority of people on the health visitor's caseload are not ill, although they will experience periods of ill-health at some time. Neither is referral to the health visitor necessarily through the medical profession. Nursing intervention in this setting is basically directed towards motivating the 'patient' to perform the required action herself. 'Patient' embodies a dependent relationship, similar to that of child and parent, whereas the working relationship sought by the health visitor is that of adult to adult. Use is made in health visiting of the word 'client' or 'family',

even in reference to one person, rather than 'patient'. This does not alter the basic character of the model or reduce its relevance as visualised by one of the co-authors. Tierney (1984) presents a broader view of nursing by looking at areas, including the community, where nursing care is not dependent on medical diagnosis. In so doing, she emphasises the relevance of the ALs over a disease model. With ALs, importance is given to promoting health, maintaining routines, and individuality, as well as following through medical treatments for disease.

Another possible difficulty lies in the use of the word 'problem'. Health visitors may well view 'patients' as having problems, but patients tend not to see this as applicable to themselves. In view of possible post-operative difficulties or age-related deterioration leading to 'problems', it may be more constructive to note how the 'patient' refers to these. Other terminology could be used and 'needs', 'topic', or 'health focus' can be substituted for 'problems'. Again this seems to be in line with how the authors view the model, for Tierney (1984) states that 'on the basis of systematically collected information a patient's nursing *needs* (commonly expressed as problems) are identified.'

Critical analysis of the AL model

The assessment of Miss Normandy's levels of independence on the ALs is shown in Figure 9.1 and Figure 9.2 represents her care plan. Actual and potential problems have been identified and validated with Miss Normandy. Because health visiting focuses strongly on the relationship built up with clients, and the skills of empathising with their needs, it was not thought appropriate always to specify behavioural goals. Instead evaluation was based on an interpretive, intuitive approach which also necessitates involvement of the client in judging whether goals have been achieved. In the care plan the 'Evaluation' column is used to record progress towards goal achievement, and here it is possible to give behavioural evidence of progress, such as 'Able to express concerns', and 'Completes transfer form'. This seems to be the most appropriate approach for health visiting, where involvement may be long-term, progress may be relatively slow, and needs may change in such a way as to make specification of firm, measurable goals difficult, if not impossible.

Several difficulties and dilemmas arose in the course of preparing these documents, connected particularly with the development of the health-visiting relationship, the question of goal-setting, and the link between these and the health visitor's own personal values and professional background. In addition the amount of documentation seemed excessive and overlaps were found between the various ALs, as others have noted (Roper *et al.* 1983).

However, using the model to guide care planning has potential benefits in terms of a more comprehensive assessment which can aid teaching and learning for both the client and the student health visitor.

In this final section the experience of writing the care plan will be critically evaluated and the emerging issues explored.

It could easily be that present habits and routines contribute towards the patient's ill health, or present a future health hazard. The health visitor would seek to modify this behaviour, over a period of time, through health education, encouragement and support. In this case, routines would be changed rather than preserved. A further interesting situation may arise, in that the patient, in full possession of the facts, disagrees with the proposed plan and resists all 'sales talk'. Compliance may be viewed as an aim of health visiting, and non-compliance seen not as a sign of the patient's self-determination but as invalidation of the health visitor's role. This can lead to a feeling of confusion for the health visitor and possible rejection of the patient. It also makes evaluation in terms of patient behaviour difficult, and in that case evaluation may be based on health visitor performance. This gives a subtle change to the meaning of evaluation, which could more accurately be termed 'justification'.

In turn, this reduces the emphasis on patient-centred care and puts more emphasis on the health visitor role. Perhaps withdrawal by the health visitor from the situation is a reasonable nursing action in some instances. It may be that the model's division into 12 areas can facilitate a continued working relationship in such circumstances, for disagreement may be in one area only, and a sizeable proportion may remain in which to find common ground and goals.

Evaluation in terms of changed patient behaviour may be difficult when working in the area of cognitive changes and in the home environment. It is impossible to evaluate preventive care accurately. A prevented event is a non-event, and it is open to question as to why it did not happen. Hargreaves (1981) discusses the fact that not all information gathered by the nurse for evaluation is measurable. Evaluation has to be based on all accessible information, both subjective and objective. This involves the fallible personal judgement of the nurse and the indefinable relationship between nurse and patient. Evaluation may often be through eliciting feedback information from the patient in an interview situation, using open-ended questions and intuitive evaluation by the nurse.

Long-term evaluation could be based on the goal of eventual resumption of all usual duties post-operatively. The variables involved, namely the surgeon's expertise, post-operative morbidity, and the effects of age, could well involve a compromise on this particular goal, with complete resumption of all activities not occurring. In this situation, the ALs allow a breakdown into specific areas in which encouragement, compromise or measurable action can be realistically evaluated.

The question of assessing potential problems also arises. This could be seen by some health visitors to occupy an excessive amount of time and to focus the patient's energies on negative events. In fact potential health hazards in the home and other areas of the patient's life are relevant topics for assessment in all visits by the health visitor. They are particularly relevant for the elderly, and are valid components of preventive health care. Research reveals that events are more predictable in an older person's life, and gives an indication of relevant health problems that are likely to occur (Gardiner 1975, Luker 1983). Hysterectomy has its own particular possible complications and in the care plan which follows potential problems are restricted to those related specifically to this.

While provision of information and equipment is within their role, many health visitors would feel that practical nursing lies outside their sphere. This issue is part of a continuing debate which questions the restrictive nature of health visiting, or conversely, the need for the Registered Nurse qualification as a basis for health visitor training. When a health visitor uses the AL model, practical nursing requirements are supplied from available community nursing resources. However, the patient may refuse the involvement of the community nurse and be unable to perform the nursing action required. There may be opposition to the use of, or even absence of, relatives or friends to help. In this event, the question arises of whether the health visitor is a possible available resource for practical help.

A criticism of the model is that it is mechanistic and that a systems approach dehumanises people, by not encouraging the patient's own coping abilities. The model, in fact, views the patient as an individual, and does allow for assessment of the patient's past coping techniques and utility of available personal resources. Use of any model is influenced by the professional background of the user as well as the user's own values (Hockey 1978). In a health visiting orientation, encouraging the patient's own coping facilities is inherent in enabling self-determination, and is a constructive use of a valuable resource.

The length of individual visits, which Luker (1983) found militated against health visitors working with older women, may at first be unchanged. More to the point, the information gained from a more structured visit validates the health visitor's role to herself in this type of visiting. It is not always necessary for all the ALs to be worked through on each visit, and the model is also conducive for use with a shortened interview schedule. This in turn may give rise to a better service to the patient and a decrease in length of visit.

Use of the ALs as a ritualistic list is a possible misuse which perhaps reflects less on the model than on the user, who may use other models in the same fashion.

When using the model, there is a possibility of inclusion of irrelevant detail, of duplication, or of omission of information. This is linked to the overlap of ALs and is another area requiring awareness and sensitivity on the part of the user.

The remaining difficulty lies in the amount of documentation, which can be time-consuming and distracting. Basically, any clerical work distracts from visiting but it is essential. If a shortened interview technique is used in subsequent visits, then the initial documentation procedure is not repeated. The extra time spent in writing notes could be viewed as an acceptable price to pay for more productive use of shorter time with the patient. On the other hand, it may also cut down job satisfaction and increase the pressures on those who view health visiting more in terms of working with people, and less as a desk-bound activity. Perhaps an answer to this problem, which exists to a degree in all methods of documentation, is for the health visitor to record her visit on an audio–cassette and then have the information typed into records by clerical staff. An alternative suggestion is to explore the idea of self-recording by the patients themselves.

Teaching implications of using the AL model

The Patient

In the learning situation, perhaps the most important factors are patient motivation and how to stimulate this. With Miss Normandy the motivation to seek out information was very strong and resulted in her approach to the health visitor.

The health visitor will seek to maintain this motivation and to extend the knowledge Miss Normandy has to other areas of her life and health. As previously stated, the model gives a clearer idea of the health visitor role and how surgery can affect the individual. Through its use Miss Normandy is enabled with the aid of diagrams, appropriate literature and discussion to learn about her body and its responses to certain stimuli. She can also be helped to prepare for and learn suitable responses to the stresses of surgery and the recovery period, such as breathing and coughing exercises. Within this learning process lie the seeds of confidence and maintenance of integrity and self-respect, and 'there is a greater chance of women being able to use information to control their own recovery in the setting of the home than in a routine-orientated hospital' (Webb 1983). Not only are coping abilities enhanced, but this positive reward which comes from learning stimulates further learning and use of resources. In this situation the preventing, comforting and seeking aspects of ALs are displayed and encouraged.

The model provides information about Miss Normandy's life-style and the opportunity to explore its effects on her health. Through its emphasis on health education, it allows her to learn and to make informed health choices, aided by the health visitor.

One very important part of assessment facilitated by the ALs is assessment of all the components required to enable the learning process to take place. These range from physical barriers, like deafness, through to cognitive factors such as motivation. Any adjustments required can then be made in order to facilitate learning. Thus the health visitor is able to treat Miss Normandy as an individual, even in the area of learning needs. Her information input can be tailored to Miss Normandy, in a style and pace that suits her. Reinforcement by books, contact with other patients, discussion, and involvement of other professionals and self-help groups can be used as appropriate.

Students

As a teaching tool for students, the model's main advantages lie in providing structure and easily understood concepts for visiting older people.

Much greater depth of relevant information is obtained and areas which might otherwise be omitted are covered by the ALs. They demonstrate need, and contribute towards the planning of individual, patient-centred care. The patient is seen as an individual influenced by all twelve dimensions of living, and this provides many teaching opportunities rather than highlighting possible failures of the health visiting role.

An example of this is the suggested change in Miss Normandy's care plan of her laundry technique. Her low economic means disbar the installation of a washing machine, or use of a commercial laundry service, but the alternative of using a launderette seems suitable until the lift breaks down. There is then a strong possibility that Miss Normandy will resume her old routine of washing laundry in the bath. This response would involve her individuality, past coping techniques, financial status, isolation and changed physical environment; the possibility illustrates the need for continuous assessment, evaluation and joint goal-setting in order to ensure that she continues to see health visiting interventions as appropriate.

For the student, difficulty in adjusting to the different orientation of health visiting in comparison with hospital nursing can be eased by use of the model. The intangible skills of the health visitor, for example interpersonal skills and establishing rapport, are made less ethereal and unexplainable through use of a conceptual framework, backed up with suitable documentation and research evidence.

The identification of relevant potential health needs through use of the model demonstrates the importance of planned preventive measures and health education, with the use of available resources. These resources include the patient's own coping processes, as well as the use of research which helps to give realistic care.

The isolation of potential areas of need allows discussion to take place before a crisis situation arises, and thereby improves the chance of successful resolution from the patient's point of view as well as the health visitor's.

Finally, documentation of the ALs, although

onerous, will provide the basis for future research and learning. Crow (1981), looking at the need for theory and concepts in research, comments that, 'If the health visitor uses her own conceptual framework, she will also see that she should not "lift" theories and apply them, but incorporate them into her own body of knowledge through the use of her own conceptual framework.' On this basis the health visitor using the process of nursing within the AL framework may be better able to use research realistically and increase her own learning.

Fig. 9.1 Assessment of Miss Normandy

A/L	Usual routine (What he/she can/cannot do independently)	Patient's problems (A) Actual (B) Potential	Goal
Maintaining a safe environment	Lives alone. Insular, no contact with immediate neighbours. Alert, active. Good understanding of home safety. No exposed fires Flat on 16th floor, lift often out of order Would like to move. Does all washing by hand in the bath	(P) Isolation, lack of care and support in post-operative period on discharge home (A) Anxiety about hospital admission (P) Difficult access at these times (A) Transfer not requested (P) Injury from bad laundry technique.	Adequate care on discharge from hospital. Support in the recovery period Adjusts to changed environment Able to cope with disruption Transfer application made Understanding of risks Safe laundry routine
Communicating	Reserved, independent lady but able to express herself verbally. Does not require glasses or a hearing aid. Is pleased to be having a hysterectomy but concerned that she doesn't know what a vaginal hysterectomy involves. Feels unable to ask the doctor questions	(A) Anxiety. Lack of information (A) Inability to use available information sources	Controllable anxiety. Knowledge about vaginal hysterectomy Uses information sources
Breathing	Does not smoke. No respiratory problems	(P) Poor respiration due to pain post-operatively. Difficulty in coughing (P) Chest infection	Control of pain. Able to cough well. Good respirations No chest infection
Eating and drinking	Limited income of pensions. Has own teeth. Cooks for self daily and for two friends twice a week. No food dislikes. Takes a balanced food intake. Prefers to drink tea. Does not drink alcohol. Not overweight	(P) Poor nutritional intake will inhibit good tissue healing (P) Weight gain or loss	Knowledge and use of good nutritional intake. Healing tissues. No weight change.
Eliminating	Dribbling, urgency and pain on micturition. Daily bowel movement	(A) Recurrent urinary infections (P) Disturbed bladder and bowel action, painful flatus post-operatively	No urinary infections Prepared for changes. Able to cope with minimal discomfort

Fig. 9.1 (continued)

A/L	Usual routine (What he/she can/cannot do independently)	Patient's problems (A) Actual (B) Potential	Goal
Personal cleansing	Clean, tidy and neatly dressed. Washes down daily. Bathes, washes hair weekly. Good hygiene with teeth and hand washing.	(P) Anxiety about changed routine (P) Wound infection	Able to adjust to changes No infection
Controlling body temperature	Dresses appropriately. Eats regular meals. Flat centrally heated.		
Mobilising	Mobile without aid. Daily walks	(A) Restricted mobility post-operatively (P) Incapacity from poor lifting techniques	Resumes daily walks Good lifting technique
Working and playing	Enjoys reading. Supports over-60's club. Shops and cooks for two separate friends twice a week. Cares for relatives when ill.	(P) Frustration at restricted activities in post-operative period	Constructive use of enforced rest. Return to normal routine
Expressing sexuality	Channels her energies into caring for others. Menopause 30 yrs ago. Does not feel that hysterectomy will make her less feminine	(P) Anxiety, guilt at 'letting people down' and needing care herself. (A) Discharge and bleeding per vaginam (A) Distaste, embarrassment at wearing sanitary towels again (P) Operation may revive regrets of life-style with no children	Able to work through feelings Arranges help for friends Prepared for temporary situation Reassertion of self-identification and self-esteem
Sleeping	Sleeps well from 11 pm–7.30 am	(P) Anxiety pre-operatively may disturb sleep	Minimal disturbance of sleep
Dying	Small fear of not waking up after anaesthetic	(P) Fear is not manageable	Able to work through thoughts Fear controllable

Fig 9.2 Care plan for Miss Normandy

A/L	Intervention	Evaluation	Date
Maintaining a safe Environment	Discuss: Care arrangements for after discharge. Possibility of staying with niece. Home Care assessment for help on return to flat.	Arrangements made for care post-operatively. Home help organiser visited and available help discussed.	2–3 weeks at next visit
	Support from local voluntary groups. Possible areas of concern from earlier stay in hospital.	Options considered and information acted on. Able to express concerns and work out possible solutions.	2–3 months In visits before admission
	Access when lift out of order.	Shows preparation, e.g. food stock, Caretaker's number obtained.	At visit
	Transfer schemes and other housing provision. Dangers of laundry routine. Offer further visits post-operatively.	Options considered. Completes transfer form Alternatives considered. Bath not used. Visit arranged and effected.	6 months 2–3 months 1–3 months post op
Communicating	Discuss: (with drawings) Vaginal hysterectomy Inability to speak to doctor. Ways to overcome this, e.g. writes questions down.	Shows understanding. Anxiety lessened. Says will follow advice through and attempts to do so.	At each visit. 2–3 weeks
Breathing	Discuss: Preparation needed before admission. Work of physiotherapist. Effect of anaesthetic. Post-operative pain relief. Good effects of daily exercise. Teach simple breathing exercises.	Shows understanding by use of questions and discussion. Continues daily walks. Does breathing exercises.	At each visit.
Eating and Drinking	Discuss: Present food intake. Any changes needed to promote healing. Effect of enforced rest on weight, appetite.	Shows understanding of nutritional requirements necessary. Controls appetite. Resumes active lifestyle. No weight change.	At each visit
Elimination	Discuss: Eliminating techniques. The effects of pelvic surgery, catheterisation, immobility and fasting on these. Helpful routines for managing effects.	Shows understanding by linking up information on vaginal hysterectomy and urinary symptoms.	At each visit

Fig 9.2 (continued)

A/L	Intervention	Evaluation	Date
Personal Cleansing and Dressing	Discuss: Difficulty in changed routine and possible compromises. Teach bowel and vulval hygiene.	Appears less anxious. Feels confident to seek aid of ward staff. Agrees its relevance.	At each visit
Mobilising	Teach lifting technique, pelvic exercises. Stress importance for post-operative period. Discuss resumption of mobility post-operatively.	Improved lifting stance. Expresses understanding.	Over next few months 6-12 weeks post-operatively
Working and Playing	Discuss: Recovery needs that restrict activities. Care options for friends.	States awareness of own needs. Shows thought and planning for this period, including arrangements for friends.	At each visit Pre-operatively
Expressing Sexuality	Discuss: Guilt feelings, importance of self value/care for well-being of carer. Validity of past achievements and life. Remind of temporary use only of pads.	Able to share feelings and use time to explore them. Rationalisation and confirmation of valid life style. Expresses tolerance.	At each visit At each visit
Sleeping	Allow time for discussion of areas of concern. Create suitable atmosphere for confidences. Achieve rapport and empathy.	Sessions are used as planned. States visits and talks have helped. Anxiety and tension less. Minimal sleep disturbance.	At each visit
Dying	Allow time to discuss fear. Encourage positive attitude.	Able to talk about and cope with fears in balance with hopes for future.	Pre- and post-operatively

References

Barker MG 1968 Psychiatric illness after hysterectomy. *British Medical Journal*, **2**, 91–95

Boore JPR 1978 *Prescription for recovery.* Royal College of Nursing, Research Series 76

Carter E 1981 Ready for home. *Nursing Times*, May 7: 826–829

Clark J 1982 A way to get organised. *Nursing Times*, Community Outlook, October 13: 287–295

Crow R 1981 Theories and concepts. *Nursing Times*, **77**, 7: 284–286

Dennerstein L, Wood C & Burrows G 1977 *Hysterectomy.* Oxford University Press, Oxford

Dicker RC, Greenspan JR, Strauss LT, Cowart MR, Scally MJ, Peterson HB, de Stefano F, Rubin GL & Ory HW 1982 Complications of abdominal and vaginal hysterectomy. *American Journal of Obstetrics and Gynecology*, **144**, 7: 841–848

Ellenborgen A, Agranat A & Grunstein S 1981 The role of vaginal hysterectomy in aged women. *Journal of American Geriatrics Society*, **29**, 9: 426–428

Feroze M 1977 Vaginal hysterectomy. *British Journal of Hospital Medicine*, **17**, 1: 69–76

Gardiner R 1975 The identification of the medical and social needs of the elderly in the community: a pilot survey. *Age and Ageing*, **4**, 3: 81–87

Goodwin MF & Steele SJ 1975 A pamphlet to answer the patient's questions before hysterectomy. *The Lancet*, September 13: 492–493

Gould D 1985 Understanding emotional need. *Nursing Mirror*, Research Forum, **160**, 1: ii–vi

Gray LA 1982 Complications of vaginal surgery. *Clinical Obstetrics and Gynaecology*, **25**, 4: 869–881

Gudex RG 1965 Pelvic floor repair with or without hysterectomy. *Journal of Obstetrics and Gynaecology of the British Commonwealth*, **72**: 864–865

Hargreaves I 1981 The nursing process. In: Smith JP (Ed) *Nursing Science in Nursing Practice.* Butterworths, London

Haslett S & Jennings M 1984 *Hysterectomy and vaginal repair.* Trustees, St Thomas' Hospital, London

Hawksworth W 1965 Indications for vaginal hysterectomy. *Journal of Obstetrics and Gynaecology of the British Commonwealth*, **72**: 847–850

Hockey L 1978 Research and the process of nursing. Paper at the RCN Research Society Annual Conference

Howkins J 1965 Vaginal and abdominal hysterectomy. *Journal of Obstetrics and Gynaecology of the British Commonwealth*, **72**: 858–860

Jones HO. & Doyle LW 1943 Studies of surgical morbidity, 1, Abdominal hysterectomy. *American Journal of Obstetrics and Gynecology*, **46**: 160

Keith C 1980 Discussion group for post hysterectomy patients. *Health and Social Work*, 1: 59–63

Kuczynski HJ 1982 After the hysterectomy. *Nursing Mirror*, August 11: 42–46

Luker KA 1983 An evaluation of health visitors' visits to elderly women. In: Wilson-Barnett J (Ed) *Nursing Research: Ten Studies in Patient Care.* John Wiley and Sons, Chichester

Morris WIC 1965 Doubts on the value of vaginal hysterectomy in the management of genital prolapse. *Journal of Obstetrics and Gynaecology of the British Commonwealth*, **72**: 860–861

Navratil E 1965 The place of vaginal hysterectomy. *Journal of Obstetrics and Gynaecology of the British Commonwealth*, **72**: 841–846

Porges RF 1980 Changing indications for vaginal hysterectomy. *American Journal of Obstetrics and Gynecology*, **2**: 153–158

Powell SR 1982 A London hospital's approach. *Nursing Mirror*, August 11: 46

Raphael B 1978 Psychiatric aspects of hysterectomy. In: Howell JG (Ed) *Modern Perspectives in the Psychiatric Aspects of Surgery.* MacMillan, London

Richards BC 1978 Hysterectomy from woman to woman. *American Journal of Obstetrics and Gynaecology*, 131, 4: 446–452

Richards DH 1973 A post hysterectomy syndrome. *The Lancet*, 2: 983–985

Roos NP 1984 Hysterectomies in one Canadian province: A new look at risks and benefits. American Journal of Public Health, *APJH* 74, 1: 39–45

Roper N 1976 *Principles of nursing.* Churchill Livingstone, Edinburgh

Roper N, Logan W & Tierney AJ 1980 *The elements of nursing.* Churchill Livingstone, Edinburgh

Roper L, Logan WW & Tierney AJ 1983 *Using a model for nursing.* Churchill Livingstone, Edinburgh

Shapiro M, Munoz A, Tager IB, Schoenbaum SC & Polk BF 1982 Risk factors of infection after abdominal or vaginal hysterectomy. *New England Journal of Medicine*, 307: 1661–1666

Sheridan MD 1973 *From birth to five years: children's developmental progress.* Windsor NFER, Nelson

Stanton SL, Hilton P, Norton C & Cardozo L 1982 Vaginal hysterectomy for prolapse. *British Journal of Obstetrics and Gynaecology*, 89, 6: 459–463

Steele SJ & Goodwin MF 1975 A pamphlet to answer the patient's questions before hysterectomy. *Lancet*, September 13: 492–493

Steptoe PC 1965 Memorandum on vaginal hysterectomy. *Journal of Obstetrics and Gynaecology of the British Commonwealth*, 72: 862–863

Stirling H 1965 Vaginal hysterectomy in the treatment of prolapse. *Journal of Obstetrics and Gynaecology of the British Commonwealth*, 72: 851–854

Tierney AJ 1984 A response to Professor Mitchell's 'simple guide to the nursing process'. *British Medical Journal*, 288: 835–838

Weaver RT 1965 Some comments on vaginal hysterectomy in Canada. *Journal of Obstetrics and Gynaecology of the British Commonwealth*, 72: 855–857

Webb A 1985 Hysterectomy counselling. *Health Visitor*, 58, 3: 61–62

Webb C 1983 A study of recovery from hysterectomy. In: Wilson-Barnett J (Ed) *Nursing Research: Ten Studies in Patient Care.* John Wiley and Sons, Chichester

Webb C 1984 Feminist methodology in nursing research. *Journal of Advanced Nursing*, 9: 249–256

Webb C & Wilson-Barnett J 1983 Self-concept, social support and hysterectomy. *International Journal of Nursing Studies*, 20, 2: 97–107

Webb C 1985 Barriers to sympathy. *Nursing Mirror*, Research Forum, 160, 1: vi–viii

Weed L 1969 *Medical records, medical education, and patient care.* Press of Cape Western University, Cleveland, Ohio

Wilson-Barnett J 1981 Recovering from illness: Looking down the road to recovery. *Nursing Mirror*, May 27: 30–33

10

Postscript

Individual authors have made critical comments both upon the models they have used as the basis for their care plans and upon the lessons learned in the process of applying the model to their own nursing care. Their experiences lead to several general conclusions which will be drawn together here.

Language

Some criticisms of nursing models may be termed 'low level' criticisms, in that they point to difficulties which are easily overcome, and several problems to do with the language used by theorists come into this category.

Whenever we start to try and come to grips with a new subject or set of ideas, we have to learn what may seem like a new language. For example, learning music involves learning new terms like crotchet and quaver, staccato and lente, bar and stave, and in the same way beginning nurse learners are at first overwhelmed by a mass of medical phraseology. To the uninitiated, the specialised terms of sociology, such as social interaction, social structure and role conflict, are often derided as meaningless and unnecessary jargon. Certainly a great deal of mystification, either unthinking or deliberate, goes on when people say 'nocte' instead of 'at night', 'upper respiratory tract infection' when they mean 'cold', and 'at this moment of time' instead of 'now'. However, when discussing abstract ideas or specialised concepts, it is essential to be precise and to use words in a way which will allow everyone involved to share the same meanings and discuss matters without confusion or ambiguity. Sometimes an upper respiratory tract infection is not simply a cold, and a chairman is sometimes a woman!

When considering the language of nursing models, we need to distinguish between the un-necessary use of roundabout ways of expressing straightforward things—for which there is no defence—and the necessary precision in defining concepts which is part and parcel of any specialised subject matter and which helps us to compare different writers' views on the same idea, such as nursing, health and patient/client. American English can often take quite a bit of unravelling, but we do not seem to find this an insurmountable problem when watching Hill Street Blues, Dallas or Dynasty! If we have the interest and will to understand, we easily sort out our initial confusions. When it comes to nursing models, however, the motivation seems to be quickly dampened; they are often rejected out of hand without trying to probe their meanings. Nothing which is rewarding in the end is likely to be easy at first, and the reflex response of many nurses when faced with the unfamiliar terminology of the models is part of a defensive anti-intellectualism which shows itself also in negative attitudes towards research in nursing and degree-level courses for nurses.

Nursing theorists have a professional obligation to make their ideas understandable to other practitioners, but nurses who aspire towards professional status have a parallel obligation to make an effort to comprehend nursing models. Writers of the care plans in this book have achieved this level of understanding, and have shown that it is possible to adapt American terminology for the British context.

Paperwork

Another 'low level' criticism of nursing models is that of the amount of documentation which seems to be required, and nurses sometimes suggest that time would be better spent on patient care than on copious paperwork.

There is certainly a potential problem in-

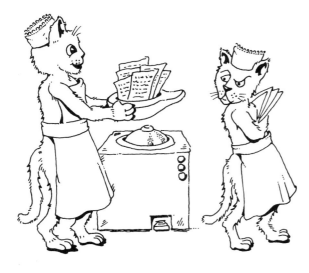

I take a very critical approach to nursing models, Sister.

volved in drawing up very detailed assessments and care plans if these have no demonstrable benefits. But it is not necessarily true that detailed documentation is a waste of nurses' valuable time, as several chapters in this book have shown. If a detailed assessment allows the nurse to detect problems in their early stages and thereby avoid serious complications, then this is time well-spent and may have cost-saving implications for the patient and health service alike. Similarly, detecting a potential problem and preventing it becoming an actual problem may save the patient from unnecessary physical, emotional and socio-economic disturbances and also lead to savings of time and money for the health service.

Another advantage of detailed assessments and care plans based on models of nursing is their use as a teaching tool with nurse learners at all levels. Trying to define measurable goals and give rationales for nursing actions in line with the model's framework can encourage an alert, thinking, critical and self-critical approach. Nurse teachers may decide that they and their students need to draw up more detailed care plans for learning purposes than are required in daily

practice. Clinical nurses need to work out how detailed assessments and care plans must be for daily practice, and whether standard care plans are a useful strategy in certain situations, such as pre- and post-operative care, or ante-natal, intra-partum and post-natal care. Several chapters in this book have illustrated the constructive use of standard care plans based on potential problems, with any actual problems which arise being transferred to an individual care plan.

The amount of detail required in a care plan is a matter for professional judgement, and the plans in this book show that it is possible to devise concise and workable plans based on models of nursing, as well as more detailed versions which lend themselves readily to a teaching context. Only by experimenting with different formats in their everyday work will nurses be able to decide what is most appropriate for them and their patients or clients, and strike a balance between the need to avoid excessive and unnecessary paperwork on the one hand and the possibility of early detection of potential or serious problems on the other hand.

Operationalising the concepts

More profound criticisms of nursing models draw attention to problems in using them because they are not spelled out in sufficient detail. Several authors in this book have found difficulty in deciding under which heading to enter a particular piece of information in an assessment scheme. This brings us back to issues raised in the introductory discussion, which questioned whether we were dealing with conceptual frameworks, models or theories. The consensus seemed to be that these terms indicated an increasing complexity and sophistication, with conceptual frameworks being the most superficial level and theories the most developed and detailed. The fact that it proves difficult or even impossible to decide how to enter information into an assessment scheme confirms that we are not dealing with fully elaborated theories of nursing. Similarly, if the goal of nursing is defined in an abstract way as 'adaptation', for example, and nursing action is left as 'manipulating stimuli' without detailed guidance about what forms adaptation or manipulation can take, then again we are working at a vague and abstract level, without complete theoretical justification for our actions. In other words, the ideas are not spelled out in a way which makes them directly translatable into action or they are not sufficiently operationalised.

Goals

The question of measurable goals proves to be a vexed one when trying to apply nursing models. Most authors in this book have struggled to produce measurable goals, accepting that it may be impossible to judge progress unless one has criteria on which to base one's judgement. But it is not always easy to do this, and sometimes the results seem artificial or a compromise, for example when specifying that the patient will *say* she is less anxious. This begs the question of what it is she might say which the nurse could accept as evidence of being less anxious. Or does the patient merely say this to please the nurse, when in fact she really still feels very anxious?

In the introductory chapter, we raised the possibility that the nursing process and recommendations to specify measurable goals may be incompatible with 'softer' nursing models including interactionist ones such as King's model. Ann Webb, in her chapter about health visiting with an older woman, concluded that there was an incongruity, and chose instead to specify broader goals which might change over time as the health visiting relationship developed and deepened. Since goals had to be negotiated with the client, and might change as the client became more accepting of the health visitor's role, it seemed a contradiction to be too explicit at the outset.

It is obviously desirable to think out clearly what we want to achieve and which are the best ways to do this, and to make these decisions jointly with patients/clients. This must be better either than ambling along with no particular objective in mind or imposing nursing decisions on patients or clients. However, nurses ought to experiment in their own practice areas with different kinds of goals in order to find the form most appropriate to their particular problems or fields of nursing. As they do this, they should ensure that the goals they decide upon are compatible with the nursing model which underlies their work.

Different model, different care?

Many writers have constructed classification schemes and lists of criteria for analysing and evaluating nursing models (see, for example, Stevens 1979, Riehl & Roy 1980, Fitzpatrick & Whall 1983, Meleis 1985). Each has designed her own scheme and highlighted different features of nursing models, resulting in complex and esoteric discussions which give little help to nurses wanting to use models as the basis for care planning. Table 10.1 is an attempt to synthesise these discussions and present a comparison of the principal ideas underlying the five models used in this book.

These comparative analyses inevitably lead us back to the question asked in Chapter 1 about the contribution of nursing models to nursing practice, and to whether their use has an influence on the quality of care given. If a nurse conceptualises a patient as having a self-care deficit, will this lead her to plan different goals and give different interventions from those she would use if she viewed the patient as maladapting or not achieving maximum independence? Will a nurse who sees her work as manipulating stimuli do different things from one who compensates for self-care deficits or enters into a process of action, reaction, interaction and transaction with patients?

We cannot answer these questions because the models are not explicit and detailed enough in their explanations of how to assess problems, devise goals, and carry out interventions. And, partly as a result of this lack of theoretical development, evaluation research has not been

Table 10.1 A comparison of the five nursing models used in previous chapters

Author	Nurse	Patient	Mode of nursing intervention	Desired outcome
Henderson	A person who assists others to carry out 14 activities of living	A person in need of assistance in carrying out 14 activities of living	Complementing and supplementing knowledge, will and strength of patient	Wholeness and independence, or peaceful death
King	Teacher, counsellor, guide, care-giver	A unique, open system/ person who is unable to meet needs for daily living or to function in roles	A process of action, reaction, interaction and transaction or sharing of perceptions	Attainment of mutually-agreed goals
Orem	Temporary self-care agent who acts for, teaches, guides, supports, or provides a supportive environment	An individual/integrated whole in need of assistance in meeting self-care needs	Wholly or partly compensatory or supportive–educative action to overcome self-care deficits	Self-care
Roper	A person who uses the nursing process to assist individuals to carry out their activities of living	A person in need of assistance in carrying out their activities of living	Promotion of independence in activities of living by means of health education, and performing preventing, comforting and (medically) dependent activities	Self-fulfillment and maximum independence
Roy	A promoter of adaptation	A person/open system who is maladapting to stimuli received from the environment	Manipulation of focal, contextual and residual stimuli	Adaptation

done to compare the efficacy of different models in practice. The care plans in this book are not systematic evaluations of the models and therefore they cannot count as evaluation research. They are instead individual nurses' attempts to experiment with the use of a model and assess its practicality and usefulness in a particular situation. Several of these nurses have found benefits in using a structured assessment which helps to avoid omissions and to detect problems which might have remained hidden and neglected if a thorough nursing history had not been taken. However, all the care plans in the book are written by experienced nurses who have specialist knowledge of the kind of care they discuss. Until rigorous testing and systematic comparisons of the models in use are carried out it will be impossible to say whether it is the individual skill, knowledge and sensitivity of a certain nurse or the use of a particular model which leads to the quality of care planned and given. Until evaluation research has been carried out we must rely on our own and others' subjective and impressionistic assessments of the benefits and difficulties associated with using nursing models.

The American experience

Nursing models have been in existence in the USA for over a decade, although they are by no means universally used there. Those who favour nursing models in the States often use one model as the philosophical basis for the entire curriculum of a nursing course or as the basis for care planning throughout a hospital. This may be linked with a quality assurance programme, as a unified approach to care by all nurses in an institution makes it easier to measure whether particular nurses or clinical areas are giving the desired standard of care. Sometimes the use of a model is combined with computerisation of care planning, so that standard care plans can be called up on a visual display unit or printed out for each patient problem identified. An individual patient's care plan then consists of an amalgam of standard plans for these problems. Standardisation and quality control may then be achieved at the cost of truly individualised patient care, and the effects on nurses' job satisfaction are at least open to question.

At the other end of the spectrum, some nurses are extremely sceptical about what, if anything, has been gained from all these years of experimenting with nursing models. Their usefulness in daily care planning is questioned, and in fact many teachers use them only with postgraduate students on masters and doctoral level courses. Among their reasons for this are the superficial understanding of basic disciplines like psychology and sociology which is evident in some models, and the obscure phraseology which they often contain (Silva & Rothbart 1984, Webb 1984).

American nurses have arrived at these judgements on the basis of their own attempts to experiment with using nursing models rather than on evidence gained from research studies. We can therefore draw few definitive lessons from their experiences, and their different culture and system of health care add further complications. But they do offer us clues and guidelines as we begin to grapple with the same issues ourselves.

Conclusion

In this book, we have reviewed and criticised the underlying basis of nursing models in general and several particular examples, using the term 'model' as a convenient label. Having examined the background to these ideas and tried to use them in practice, we can now draw some conclusions about their intellectual status.

The full, detailed development and operationalisation required of a theory was found to be lacking. The models have generally not been empirically tested and indeed are probably not empirically testable in their present forms, precisely because they are not elaborated in sufficient detail.

Several models have been shown to incorporate conflicting philosophical and methodological ideas, probably resulting from insufficient understanding by their authors of the models and theories of other disciplines (e.g. psychology and sociology) from which they are drawn. Nursing 'models' in existence at present are therefore no more than the 'private images' (Fawcett 1984) of their originators, and are based on philosophies and assumptions which individual nurses may or may not find compatible with their own personal philosophies of life and of nursing.

This leaves several choices open to us as nurses. We could simply reject these approaches as bases for practice because of their inadequacies. But in doing this we would have to acknowledge that all practice is based on personal value choices, whether we make these explicit or not. In the past, nursing practice has been based on the medical model, and if we reject these nursing approaches we may well fall back into using that again. If we wish to reject both the medical model and the nursing approaches so far developed, then we must build our own.

Alternatively, we can accept existing nursing approaches for what they are, namely philosophies which can serve as guidelines, loose frameworks or approaches to nursing. At this level, they can serve as useful checklists which help to ensure that we have a systematic and structured way of planning and giving care.

If we decide to use existing approaches in this way, we have two further options. Either we can choose a version on the basis of its suitability to a particular individual patient or type of nursing (such as medical, psychiatric or community nursing), or we can adopt the approach which fits most comfortably with our own personal philosophy of life and of nursing, as Fawcett (1984) suggests. However, it is not clear how these strategies could be translated into practice. It is hard to envisage how several nurses in a ward, for example, would each use a different and personally acceptable approach, just as it is difficult to see how each patient could be nursed using a model suited to her but different from that used with others in the same ward. On the other hand, it seems too restricting and contrary to the notion of individualised patient care to impose one approach on a whole hospital or nurse education programme in the interests of standardisation, as is often the case in the USA (Riehl & Roy 1980, Fawcett 1984).

As yet, then, the problems of theoretical thinking about and for nursing have no easy solutions. The approaches we have at present are in many ways deficient and unsatisfactory, but probably they must be the basis for future progress simply because they are all we have. Our role as nurses seeking to carry out our work in a rational and constructively critical way is to analyse and experiment with them, and to adopt, reject or modify them using informed judgement and sound reasoning. We hope that, like the critical theorist described in Chapter 1, our efforts in this book make a contribution towards helping nurses to

> actively engage in deciding what it is they want, and what arrangements must be altered or established to fulfill themselves.
>
> (Fay 1975: 105)

References

Fawcett J 1984 *Analysis and evaluation of conceptual models of nursing.* FA Davis, Philadelphia

Fay B 1975 *Social theory and political practice.* George Allen & Unwin, London

Fitzpatrick J & Whall A 1983 *Conceptual models of nursing. Analysis and application.* Robert J Brady Co, Bowie, Maryland

Meleis AI 1985 *Theoretical nursing: development and progress.* JB Lippincott, Philadelphia

Riehl JP & Roy C 1980 *Conceptual models for nursing practice.* Appleton-Century-Crofts, New York

Silva MC & Rothbart D 1984 An analysis of changing trends in philosophies of science on nursing theory development and testing (sic). *Advances in Nursing Science*, 6, 2: 1–13

Stevens BJ 1979 *Nursing theory. Analysis, application, evaluation.* Little, Brown, Boston

Webb C 1984 On the eighth day god created the nursing process – and nobody rested. *Senior Nurse*, 1, 33: 22–25

Index